Discover the Joy of Good Health

Southwest Tennessee Community College
Gill Center Library
3833 Mountain Terrace
Memphis, TN 38127

GILL CENTER LIBRARY

DISCOVER THE JOY OF GOOD HEALTH

John Inzerillo, M. D.

Humanics Publishing Group
Atlanta, GA • Lake Worth, FL

Humanics Publishing Group

Discover the Joy of Good Health
© 2012 by John Inzerillo, M.D.
A Humanics Publishing Group Publication
First Edition

No part of this book may be reproduced or transmitted in any form or by any means, electronic or mechanical, including photocopying, recording, or by any other information storage and retrieval system, without written permission from the publisher. For information, contact:

Humanics Publishing Group
PO Box 1608
Lake Worth, FL 33460
USA
Humanicspub.com
email: Humanics@mindspring.com

Humanics Publishing Group and its trademark, consisting of the words "Humanics Publishing Group" is registered in the U.S. Patent and Trade-mark Office and in other countries.

Printed in the United States of America and the United Kingdom

ISBN (Paperback) 978-0-89334-864-9

Library of Congress Cataloging-in-Publication Data

Inzerillo, John.
Discover the Joy of Good Health / John Inzerillo. -- 1st ed.
p. cm.
Includes bibliographical references.
ISBN 978-0-89334-864-9 (pbk.)
1. Health--Psychological aspects. 2. Health attitudes. 3. Interpersonal relations. 4. Mind and body. I. Title.
R726.5.I65 2012
613--dc23
2012022690

Dedicated to my wife Treva and boys John & Joel

TABLE OF CONTENTS

Introduction 1

Chapter 1 | A Genuine Smile 7

Chapter 2 | Point of Focus 23

Chapter 3 | Praise Your Perfection 39

Chapter 4 | Conditions We Live By 53

Chapter 5 | How to Study Compassion 75

Chapter 6 | Changing Views 101

Chapter 7 | Who's in Charge 121

Chapter 8 | The Art of Doing Nothing 143

Chapter 9 | Joy 4 You 163

Summary 179

INTRODUCTION

Ever take the time to think about how you appear to others? It's easy to put on a mask that tells others to keep their distance, yet doing so keeps us apart from the rest of the world. Think for a moment of what it would feel like to be truly present, content, basking and relaxing, wearing an energizing, radiant smile, feeling as comfortable, cozy, and composed as a young kitten softly purring, seated on a pillowed dormer on a lazy, rainy day.

Have you ever wondered how you could do less and achieve more? *Discover the Joy of Good Health* will remind you of forgotten ways of opening your heart to yourself and others. It will remind you of the power of patience and the strength behind a simple smile. By following your forgiving nature you will recognize latent virtues and buried strengths. In the cultivation of personal honesty and sincerity you will develop pictures of health that will guide you toward the manifestation of your dreams.

In life we all help each other. We are all mirrors for each other, reflecting back words, images, attitudes, and actions. Through focus and presence there can be greater connectedness of intentions, emotions, and feelings as we look for opportunities to express old ideas in creative and novel ways. By living in a creative spirit, recognizing the temporary nature of all things, and accepting grace as an antidote for shortcomings, we soften and make space for ourselves and our relationships. With the activation of imagination we can learn to be grateful in all things and recognize what we have to offer in our transformation.

Good music, plays, and acts of kindness allow us to appreciate the value of others. As we are inspired in the presence of perfection, the power of authentic praise shows us the loving and caring sides of ourselves. To appreciate our changing needs opposites are necessary, as a quality or virtue cannot be fully learned without understanding its opposite. We cannot not appreciate happiness without knowing grief, and in the intimacy our own sadness we can lift up others when they are down.

We can only give true praise through our connections with others. In contributing to the welfare of others we integrate our individual sub personalities and realize the learning curve that we are all on. Remembering that we are all a work in progress allows us to live in a state of continual grace and forgiveness. Our good health depends on the appreciation of others. In addition appreciating the wondrous, spontaneous workings of our minds and bodies paves the way for authentic praise that elevates others as well as us.

Everyone is capable of mindful and intentional action. However, when external forces act as primary motivators we get lost, wasting time spinning our wheels, and tend to repeat past behaviors with the expectation of getting different results. As we experiment and work at becoming salesmen for our imaginations we begin to make friends with uncertainty. Daily as we learn more and more on how to take care of ourselves we can trust that we will find unconditional peace. As you become familiar with your own pictures of health as you read this book, many aspects of your life will come into balance and a sense of contentment will predominate.

While reading through the book readers are encouraged to give up their struggles, drop the drama from their lives, and expand their consciousness by discovering compassion through the transformation of suffering. As this happens one is able to practice genuine communication to convey today's needs to others. Readers will notice that their modus operandi becomes one of concern for the welfare of others and decision making shifts to include choices that benefit all concerned. The chapter on practicing compassion will take readers through a ten-point scale so that a daily compassion assessment can be calculated and cultured.

If you start questioning yourself as to why one would take on the study of compassion, a straight-forward answer is that it transforms anger and fear into acceptance and peace.

Over the years I have heard that in life there are two things that are certain: death and taxes. In my readings and study I can add a third certainty—change. Many are adverse to change because it forces us to think differently; it takes us out of our comfort zones. When we begin to make the connection that all change depends on the choices we consciously or unconsciously make, we can stop complaining, as complaining is a trap that keeps us from adapting to inevitable change.

Authority issues center around the concepts of trust versus fear. To find what it is that needs to manifest in your life it is necessary to dig deeply within to find the voice of wisdom. The voice may be hidden behind depression and despair. If so, you have to touch these feelings to get through them. At times we have to give ourselves permission to be the best that we can be. No one or no circumstance can keep you from your desired good. In working with authority issues the main goal is to overcome your own resistance to listening to your inner voice.

In uncertain times the best action may be to just sit and do nothing. Yet when you think about it, we can never really do nothing. But intentionally quieting the mind allows you to evaluate all of your options. What activities fill your day and how do they compare with the average American? Data from 2010 tells us that Americans are watching more TV than ever. In addition, women are spending five hours less per week on leisure time than men, telling us that women are getting more caught up in the work world. Less time for leisure equates to less time for contemplation. On the other hand, doing nothing creates space that allows us to drop past concerns and prevents us from jumping ahead to future potential roadblocks. In nothingness, we may find contentment that opens the door to forgiveness and healing.

In August 2011, Hurricane Irene left much of the East Coast without power for days. On that first evening without power, the dark was actually quite welcome as my wife and I watched our boys play board games together by candlelight instead of having their heads buried in their video games.

What brings you joy? Looking at old family photos is one way to rekindle a sense of joy. Both joy and sorrow are transient emotions, but we have the capacity to generate joy by doing the things we love. We can minimize sorrow by keeping our mind focused on joy. Appreciating the successes of others is an often overlooked way of bringing joy into your life, as is being thankful in everything that you have now, especially so if you have your health.

Instead of being anxious or nervous about the future, it is easy to rename your feelings as being "excited about the future," optimistically looking forward. In the state of joy we find a place where we can clearly see more options and potential. Removing ourselves from the roots of suffering, dropping negative expectations, and accepting the present, we can know that we are each capable of re-creating ourselves and optimizing our health in each new moment. We each have the power to make the right choices when we *Discover the Joy of Good Health*. My wish for you is that each day you take the time to make the right choices for yourself.

CHAPTER 1

A Genuine Smile

As your awareness grows and your attention begins to move away from self-centeredness, you will occasionally notice an individual or two who exhibits a beaming smile and radiates attractive energy.

What it is that drew your attention to them? Surely we have all seen people smile and express happiness before. On closer examination you see that their facial muscles are soft, the forehead skin is smooth and unruffled, there is an obvious absence of squinting, and the entire body looks relaxed and free. Their hands move with flowing grace, occasionally gesturing to add emphasis to their words. Even though you cannot hear what they are saying, you continue watching and wonder what it is that makes them shine. Looking around you may notice others who are antsy, their eyes darting from side to side, looking on alert. If you are deeply aware, you pick up the scent of their anxiety which is openly advertised by frowns and deeply furrowed brows. On the other hand, the smiling person is calm, peaceful, relaxed, and present. Why is that, you wonder? This individual is comfortable with who they are and their soul is at ease in the present.

Anatomists know that it takes 17 facial muscles to smile and 43 to frown.[1] So who is expending greater energy—the happy person or the distraught one? Of the 600 voluntary muscles in the body, the strongest one is the *masseter* muscle. The major function of this muscle is to raise the lower jaw in preparation for chewing, but it also functions to clench the teeth. It is activated in any state associated with anger or aggression.[2] We are all aware of these dark emotions, but not everyone is able to view them as useful energies. Anger, when managed and directed appropriately, can be used to help us achieve our goals. The energy behind the anger can keep us mobilized when at other times we would just give up. Aggression will also keep us on task as we will not be easily swayed to change course when things do not seem to be going our way. Michael Douglas, the actor well-known for his roles in *Romancing the Stone, Fatal Attraction, Wall Street*, and many other successful movies, was noted to say that he is such a convincing actor because he knows how to direct and use his anger on the stage.

On the other hand, unprocessed anger and aggression leads to chronic tension in the masseter muscle, thus leading to such conditions as *bruxism* (grinding of the teeth while sleeping) and *temporalmandibular joint dysfunction*, or TMJ (pain...). These conditions, with the chronic contraction of muscles, wear you out even when you are asleep. You awaken in the early hours of the morning feeling just as tired as you where when you went to bed. This, as we all know, is not a good way to start the day.

Individuals attempting to smile while they suffer from any of the above conditions will demonstrate a false smile. The energy behind the smile is forced. The nose is crunched up between the eyebrows, the teeth are clenched, and the masseter muscles are protruding visibly from the sides of the cheeks. In some instances the masseters are twitching. When a person is pressured, the neck muscles are tense and firmly contracted because these long band-like muscles respond in a field-like effect to the tension in the facial muscles. In a tense state, it is easy to wonder why others are not as friendly to us as we are trying to be with them. The forced nature of the smile counteracts the conditions necessary for awareness and keeps us separate and apart from others. The forced smile keeps us away from true presence.

An interesting two-minute exercise to try is to find a picture of yourself when you were 2 to 5 years old. See if you can find one where you are the only person in the photo. Use a picture that shows you standing, sitting, or playing alone. Ideally look for a picture where you are out in nature, at a local park or at the beach. Make sure the picture shows you looking at the camera but not to the degree that you are stiffly posing. Try to find one that shows you in a natural state. First look at the shine in your eyes. Notice the wonder, joy, deep contemplation, and presence expressed by your eyes. See that person as the picture of health that he or she was back then.

Thich Nhat Hanh, in his book *no Death, no Fear,* tells us that we are that same person, then again we are not.[3] This paradox helps us understand that though we are aging and slowing down, sagging in places we'd rather not talk about, balding and graying, and getting grumpier with the passage of time, we still possess the characteristics of innocence, appreciation and goodness. The condition of time has changed our appearance, yet our childhood has made us the adult we are today.

Can you look at that picture and take that child into your heart? Can you hold and hug him and tell him that you love him? Do not back away and try to explain anything to yourself. Simply be with the person you used to be. Feel the connection between who you were and who you are now. The link was never broken. It has only been forgotten. You are capable of remembering it at all times, allowing your words and actions to express just what that child was feeling.

In the picture, if you look deeply, you will see that the child was not separate from his surroundings. The trees in the background, the grass under his feet, the light grey boulder to his right, and the blue in the sky were all there. All there, together at the same time, these images were frozen in time by the magic of photography.

Those who remain frozen are the ones with the false smiles, while those who remain awake in the moment, and who have allowed themselves to feel as they grew, are those blessed with true smiles. They are the ones who feel joy when there is joy to be felt. They feel pain when there is pain because they do not fear pain and because they know that even pain is temporary. Anger does not put fear into their hearts as they know that anger, too, is a legitimate yet transient emotion.

Let us not be satisfied with a superficial examination of the genuine smile and its source. Those who are truly genuine experience what Thomas Moore explains in his book, *Dark Nights of the Soul*: "The dark night saves you from being stuck in your small life. It makes you a hero. It grows you into your fate and into being a responsive member of your community. In your mother's womb you were becoming a person. In your womb-like dark night you are becoming a soul."[4]

When you know who you are, you can smile when you are moved to smile. If you have lived and survived by trying to please others or by trying to be a good person all of the time, you cannot understand what it feels like to really smile or to feel joy. It simply takes too much effort and energy to keep the mask on. If you find that you are one of the "false people," this is the first step in making changes. This is not the time to tell yourself that this is all baloney. If you do, you will remain as lost as you are now. It is wiser to say that maybe some of this makes sense and open yourself up to, if not a new way of thinking, another way of seeing things.

This is the time to ask: What happened to that smile? What events, thoughts, and ideas, wiped that smile from that young face? Was it a matter of being too hard on yourself without letup, or having too many high expectations of yourself by not allowing yourself to make healthy mistakes from which you could learn? This is not the time to get angry and make excuses as to why things are the way they are for you today, but it is the time to look objectively at what happened.

Another good exercise to aid in the unfolding of events is to sit down and take the next twenty minutes to construct a time line of your life. Start with your earliest memory. You may want to go through your family photo albums, if they are still available to you, for clues. On your time line list your age, the year, and any events you recall. On a separate sheet of paper list each event and write down the specifics as to what you were feeling as these events occurred. Be as honest as possible and you will probably find that many of your feelings were ambiguous. For example, when your parents brought home your new brother or sister for the first time, you may have been absorbed in the joy of the moment as everyone oohed and aahed over the little one, and at the same time maybe you began to feel dethroned. You no longer commanded the attention you sought and so enjoyed.

After you have written down the mixture of feelings you experienced, in another column write your true feelings. If anger was one of them then accept it. As an adult you can understand how a child can all of a sudden feel left out. Jealousy, anger, doubt, and fear are real emotions. If you were lucky, an adult (or your parents) would have come to you and explained that you were still loved. They would have explained that just because the little one is so needy, it doesn't mean that you are now forgotten. In a healthy family, the next to the youngest actually moves up in rank and assumes the role of the older sibling, who will eventually help the younger sibling learn the ropes of childhood. This kind of reassurance leads to genuine smiles by all.

Today, you have the ability to go back to the child in the picture and clarify what the reality of the time was. Imagination is a powerful tool. Now is the time to use it as the child inside is ready to listen. For so long he has been crying to be heard. Speak to him with gentleness; explain the situation until all the misunderstanding has been erased, and then with a genuine smile, open your arms to him as you give him all of the love that you have. Watch as he smiles and beams back to life.

Probably the most famous smile in the world is that of Leonardo da Vinci's *Mona Lisa*.[5] Based on the Ekman and Friesen's Facial Action Coding System which codes for different types of smiles, her smile is a simple smile.[6] This smile involves only raising the corners of the lips. Her lip and facial features bring to mind the image we are instructed to hold when in a state of meditation. As Richard Rosen tells us in *Yoga Breathing*,[7] while following the breath in Buddhist meditation, in our minds eye, we are to wear an inner smile. This is useful even if you do not necessarily feel like smiling because the intention activates the muscles involved in smiling and the mind responds by triggering past happy memories. In a sense you are fooling your mind into thinking you are happy. Mona Lisa's mysterious smile appears to have a hidden meaning also, as scientists believe it to be a self-portrait of Leonardo.

Marsilio Ficino, a fifteenth-century Florentine scholar and philosopher, guided and advised his followers on ways to reconnect with the knowledge of their own souls.[8] In Letter 28, Ficino writes to Lorenzo de' Medici (the grandson of Cosimo de' Medici who was the patriarch of one of the wealthiest families, and thus patron of the arts during the Italian Renaissance) the following: "The soul is not satisfied by mortal things, for it seeks again the eternal."[9] In this letter, Ficino tells Medici that "we all thirst for the good and the true, yet we all drink dreams."[10] Ficino has figured out what we all know, but what many of us fail to do: that is to appreciate what is within ourselves and stop looking for happiness and satisfaction from outside sources. Ficino writes that we need to turn our thinking around and reorient our motivations by 180 degrees. This message is brought home in the following passage:

"What therefore is to be done, so that we may be of good strength and good vigilance? Life for us should straightway be turned right round in the opposite direction. Those

things which we have learned from the many should be unlearned; in having to learn which, we have up to now ignored our own selves. Those things left undone should be learned; the which having been ignored, we cannot know ourselves. What we neglect should be esteemed; what we esteem should be neglected. What we flee from, should be borne; what we pursue should be fled. For us the smile of fortune should bring tears; and the tears of fortune should bring a smile. For by these means, the filth of the multitude will not defile us, nor will the carelessness of immortal things harm us, nor desire for knowledge of mortal things torment us."

It appears that those who, in fact, do show us genuine smiles are the individuals who have been able, in one way or another, to experience their true nature. Those who are fortunate have had such attitudes passed down from one generation to the next. Others have had to struggle to come to terms with the meaning of their lives, living the best that they could from moment to moment, making mistakes, learning from their mistakes, and starting over time and time again. The healthy attitude here seems to be a paradox as most of life is. Those who intrinsically know their own worth, and who function day to day based on their beliefs also know and understand that they have been blessed by the grace of God. They who find the most enjoyment in life are those who understand these things, and they are the ones who smile with ease and comfort.

It is as if the person who offers a genuine smile is willing to give more of themselves to others. As reported by Vijai P. Sharma, Ph.D., a study was performed to assess the correlation between a genuine smile and happiness in life. Psychologists reviewed smiles found in a college yearbook and divided them into "Duchenne" smiles, considered to be genuine smiles (smiles that curl up the corners of the mouth and generate crow's feet-like folds around the eyes), and "perfunctory," or courtesy smiles. All smilers were contacted at age 27, 43, and 52 and were asked about the health of their marriage and their overall satisfaction in life.

The women with the genuine smiles were more likely to be married and remain married as well as being more likely to have a greater sense of well-being. These results held up over a thirty-year period and had nothing to do with overall attractiveness. It seems that these individuals were the ones with stable feelings of joy and cheerfulness.[11]

This is all well and good for those individuals with a genetic predisposition to being cheerful and happy (the role of genetics is reported to be as high as 80% as studied in middle-aged twins)[12], but what does this mean for those who say they are just not happy? Such statistics bring us back to the nature/nurture controversy or the proverbial "which came first: the chicken or the egg?" What is necessary for those who were born without a genetic predisposition for happiness is to follow the path of their inner voice and accept their current condition, make friends with who they are, and through self-study and self-reflection, determine what they want to change, if anything.

Philip Martin in *The Zen Path through Depression* tells us the following: "What may be crucial to our healing is, first, to do nothing.[13] When you are burdened with disease, such as the physical maladies that are so prevalent like arthritis, difficult-to-control diabetes, any type of debilitating heart disease such as a cardiac arrhythmia, angina, or congestive heart failure, or any of the known cancers, of which lung, breast, colon, and prostate are the most common, it is almost impossible to show the world a true smile since these disease states are so taxing on the individual. Many of my patients come in and tell me that since their diagnosis of cancer every little thing they notice that is different in their body triggers a response in them that leads them to think, "Oh my God, the cancer is back."

Individuals who suffer from psychological conditions such as depression, anxiety, obsessive-compulsive disorder, or bipolar disorder, to name a few, also are running on empty. It is as if their conditions keep them at the lowest levels of Maslow's Hierarchy of Needs. They are always functioning in survival mode. The smiles we see on their faces are of nervous origin, or of attempting to be polite.

When Pema Chodron tells us to meditate using the method of *tonglen*, or sending and taking, she instructs us that we are to do so with an open heart. First we have to touch our own pain and shortcomings and get comfortable with our own demons. Once this is accomplished we can wish for others to, "know happiness and the root of happiness."[14] What exactly is the root of happiness? What will allow all of us to express our genuine smiles most of the time? Some reports will tell you that confidence is what makes you smile. According to a report in *USA Today*, the USA is the third happiest country in the world, ranking between first and fourth in eight of the ten happiness categories. For Americans, their greatest source of happiness is related to the level of self-confidence. For most of the 1990s, Americans have become more self-reliant, more optimistic, and are feeling better about themselves.[15]

On the surface, it may seem that the root of happiness is different for each individual, though many would have themselves believe that money is the root of happiness. Delving deeper into the question shows that desire for possessions can never lead to lasting happiness. Holding such beliefs is like drinking water one time and thinking that you will never have to drink again. Go five days without water and see how you feel. By then you would give everything you own for a drink of water. The ability to see clearly is closer to what will make you happy. The knowledge of your intrinsic goodness and your ability to love and be loved is what makes you genuine. Until you begin to accept these ideas, your smiles will continue to look like paint on cardboard. You are fooling no one except yourself.

If you find that you are living ahead of yourself, thinking that things will be wonderful and perfect when you achieve a certain goal or when your bank account reaches a predetermined number, then you are living from the outside. When you are ready to make a change and start living with the intention to begin the process of unveiling yourself to yourself, one of the first steps to take is to choose the virtues that you want to live up to. When you get up in the morning and tell yourself that you will intentionally express compassion for everyone you come into contact for the next sixteen hours, all of the petty concerns of your yesterdays and tomorrows will vanish. You will no longer care who makes more money than you, or who has better looks than you, or even who may appear smarter than you. Your goal will be to open your heart to all people regardless of their station or circumstances.

As you exercise the power of such intention you will find that you no longer come home from work feeling exhausted. You find that you do not get angry as often as you had, and when you do express anger it is over something that truly makes you angry. The beauty of this is that you will know this and the anger will no longer stop you from feeling, but will help you understand your part in what is going on around you. It can also give you the opportunity to initiate needed changes that will not only affect your corner of the world but also the lives of others.

In his bestselling book, *The 7 Habits of Highly Effective People*, Stephen R. Covey uses the idea of principles instead of virtues. Some of the principles that he discovered being used by highly effective people included fairness, integrity, honesty, human dignity, service, quality, potential, growth, patience, nurturance, and encouragement. Instead of living on the level of personalities, he suggests new levels of thinking which are principles centered.[16]

In making your decision to take the difficult steps to uncovering your authentic self, you need to feed and water your patience. You need to nurture and encourage yourself especially through the negative self-talk that will make itself known once you make your decision to change. A forgiving attitude will go a long way in bringing you to a proactive position as you see where you have allowed yourself to get stuck in the past. Know that such lack of forward movement was due to personal ignorance of the virtues that you have possessed all of your life. Drop the guilt, give up on blaming anyone else for your lack of progress, and put your energies into fully expressing your unique virtues. If you do this, one day you will wake up and find yourself smiling, and know that it is the real thing.

As we all know, not all smiles indicate happy thoughts. Smiles can be used to show reassurance, amusement, and ridicule. They can also be used to mask other emotions, especially insecurity. A smile can turn a tense situation into a more comfortable situation. The associated facial expressions and body language you display when smiling can also be used to express aggression, sarcasm, and other negative emotions.[17]

John Inzerillo, M. D.

Take a few moments and review your day. For as many encounters with others as you can recall, think about the smiles that you shared today. Which ones were genuine and backed by a real connection with others? How did it feel to give such a smile? Did you notice that your personal worries vanished momentarily while you were smiling? Now recall the smiles expressed while you were in a tense situation or while you were under pressure to perform? Thinking on these things, can you feel the heaviness associated with the nervous smile as compared to the openness and lightness experienced with the genuine smile?

Let's examine this a bit deeper and look to see what your need to smile was during the moments of stress. Was it an attempt to take attention away from a perceived character deficiency in yourself, or a way of asking for acceptance from others because you did not have a ready answer to their question or questions? What would have been a more honest response on your part, and if you had chosen to respond in that way, how would you have felt differently?

By examining your habitual responses to all of your encounters you can rewrite and voice over your old responses and act from your genuine self. When you do this, your sense of self-respect will expand and the change will be noticed by those in your circles. Do not make this a more difficult examination than it is by adding self-judgment or criticism. Make it a friendly inner conversation where your higher self suggests to you where you can make small but positive changes in your attitude. The behavioral change will follow the inner change. If you decide to be more honest and sincere with yourself, the result will be less inner conflict and greater peace. In being honest you drop the need to defend yourself.

Donald DeMarco, in *The Heart of Virtue: Lessons from*

Life and Literature Illustrating the Beauty and Value of Moral Character tells us that the word "sincere" comes from the Latin *sincerus,* which means "sound", "whole", "pure", "genuine", or "unmixed".[18] He notes that which we already know: people like and are attracted to individuals who are open and sincere. Those who know themselves are able to be themselves and come across as real. On the other hand, one's inner struggles are also obvious to those who care to take note. Such inner conflict is broadcast to all by posture, choice of words, congruence of speech and thought, appropriateness of response to others words and conditions, and general affect. In order to live in health and project a healthy affect, sincerity alone is not enough. It must be combined with a genuine interest in others, as well as a deep understanding of your own potential, and a realistic recognition of your limitations. As wisdom is gained through experience and reflection, a genuine appreciation of self will manifest. Only then will the inner smile be true. When this is the case there is no reason to fake anything or pretend to be someone you are not.

Notes: A Genuine Smile

1. From Body Teen.com. *Anatomy* http://www231.pair.com/grpulse/bt/anmufa.html
2. From Masseter Muscle of the Face. http://face-and-emotion.com/dataface/expression/masseter.html
3. Tich Nhat Hahn, n*o Death, no Fear* (New York: Riverhead Books, 2002), pp. 27-28.
4. Thomas Moore, *Dark Nights of the Soul* (New York, Gotham Books, 2004), p. 13.
5. A picture of the Mona Lisa can be viewed at the following web-site: http://www.paris.org/Musees/Louvre/Treasures/gifs/Mona_Lisa.jpg
6. The different types of smiles as described by psychologists today are explained in: "New perspectives on smiles and their role in positive emotions." The was from a symposium chaired by Daniel S. Messinger and can be reviewed at: http://www.isisweb.org/ICIS2000Program/web_pages/group346.html
7. Richard Freeman, Yoga Breathing: Guided Instructions on the Art of Pranayama. Sounds True. soundstrue.com.
8. From the introduction of *Meditations on the Soul: Selected Letters of Marsillio Ficino,* translated from the Latin by members of the Language Department of the School of Economic Science, London. First published in the United States of America 1996, Rochester, Vt. Introduction by Clement Salaman.
9. Ibid., page 48.
10. Ibid., page 48.
11. Vijai P. Sharma, *A Genuine Smile Goes a Long Way*. Cited from Mind Publications: http://www.mindpub.com/art458.htm.
12. D. Lykken, and A. Tellegen. May 1996. Happiness Is a Stochastic Phenomenon. *Psychological Science* 7:3:pp.186-89.
13. Phillip Martin, *The Zen Path through Depression* (SanFrancisco, Harper, 1999), p. 1.
14. Pema Chodron, *Start Where You Are: A Guide to Compassionate Living* (Boston, Shambhala, 1994). This is a guidebook that shows readers how to develop "the courage to work with our own inner pain and discover joy, well-being, and confidence."
15. From an article entitled *Happiness is the American Way: Confidence, not money, makes us smile. That, plus good sex.* USA Today, 12/13/99. Cited from http://sq.4mg.com/NationHappiness.htm
16. Stephen R. Covey, *The 7 Habits of Highly Effective People: Powerful Lessons in Personal Change* (New York, Simon & Schuster, 1989), pp. 34-44.
17. Cited from Professional Polish *Star Quality Newsletter*, Nov.2003: http://www.professional-polish.com/nl/nov03/.
18. Donald DeMarco, *The Heart of Virtue: Lessons from Life and Literature Illustrating the Beauty and Value of Moral Character* (San Francisco, Ignatius Press, 1996), pp. 208-211.

CHAPTER 2

Point of Focus

To get a clear picture a camera needs to be in focus. Now that we have digital cameras with higher and higher resolution, focusing is more a function of pixel power. When the mind is focused we enjoy the benefits of greater clarity and life seems easier. As we raise our consciousness through mindfulness training, our ability to focus sharpens. Mindfulness is a type of meditation that essentially involves focusing your mind on the present. To be mindful is to be aware of your thoughts and actions in the present, without judging yourself. On the other hand, those who suffer from Attention Deficit Disorder (ADD) find it difficult to complete assigned tasks, as their concentration and focus are relatively scattered. All complicated tasks require a degree of concentration and focus to complete, and looking at how complicated life can be, it makes sense to want to be able to focus your attention on demand.

The *Star Wars* movies brought the power of lasers to the forefront. Twenty-five years after its debut you can still go to Walmart and buy a toy light saber. My four year old has one. A laser works because it has the following properties: 1) the wave length of light is monochromatic (has one specific color) that is determined by the amount of energy released when the electron drops to a lower orbit, 2) the light is organized, and 3) it is tightly focused, concentrated, and directional. Bringing these characteristics together requires a process called *stimulated emission*. This means that all of the electrons released are in the same excited state. Another requirement for laser function is the presence of a pair of mirrors. *Photons*, or packets of light, bounce back and forth between the mirrors resulting in a cascade effect, stimulating other electrons to drop down an orbit to spin with electrons of similar wave length. The beam is concentrated to such a degree that the power of the laser is sharp and precise.[1]

You do not have to be well-versed in the physics of lasers to realize that when your mind works with focus you are capable of accomplishing more than anticipated in less time. When you experience these moments you are in a state of what Mihaly Csikszentmihalyi calls "flow".[2] There are ways to connect to this state that will be reviewed in detail later, but if your energy is all wrapped up in scattered thoughts and over-excitement, without a sense of direction, your power dissipates. Your motor is running without the benefit of traction to the wheels, thus you come up short of your goals. The increased effort fails to yield your desired result and you are left wondering what you could have done differently. It is actually a good thing to ask yourself how things could have been done differently, as long as you eventually act on your revelations. These behaviors need to be recognized as you redirect your energies toward positive outcomes.

We as individuals also act as mirrors for each other, always attentive to how others respond to our words and actions. As we live by the Golden Rule we reap the same. Treating others with respect and kindness brings us closer to our true nature. Such behavior helps us attract what we need, even though we may not know exactly what that is in the moment. Living a self-centered existence brings many hours of loneliness instead of renewing solitude. Attitudes and actions affect everyone in our circle. The choice to move from a positive perspective allows us to connect with the goodness and highest in others. Each moment that passes brings us another opportunity to choose what is best for us and those in our circle. We need to pray and meditate for the wisdom to make the best choices. As we feel more comfortable with ourselves we allow others to be themselves. The curtain of expectations drops and a sense of ease becomes the point of focus.

Mindfulness, or intentional awareness, keeps your attention focused on the task at hand. It awakens you from the sleep of ignorance as you enhance the connection between your intentions, emotions and feelings. In this context you ideally remain between full concentration and not being too hung up on the end result. Tasks are performed for the simple pleasure of doing them. Since you are not tied to any particular outcome, there is no ground for disappointment.

The trick is to enjoy the process and take the work out of achieving your goals. When you derive satisfaction from what you do, the soil is fertile for expressing creativity. By dropping fixed concepts, new avenues of thinking arise as you connect old ideas in novel ways. These connections make it easier to direct your effort toward your desires. Why relinquish precious moments that can never be reclaimed in an unfocused state, when you can choose to be mindful and direct your own way?

We are connected and engaged when we choose to open to our creative spirit. It is satisfying to spend time in activities exercising full awareness and bringing new ideas to light. The act of creation is an outlet for the emotions of anger and rage. Transformation occurs when there is a burning desire for change. This inner shift happens when you view yourself as a witness to your thoughts and not the expression of your thoughts.[17] Accepting these ideas and moving toward creative self-expression readjusts your point of focus and puts new meaning into life by allowing you to be a part of something bigger than yourself.

Regardless of what you have to do, you can choose to be mindful and aware. To do so places the power back in your hands, where it belongs. The options are to continue on a fearful path, or accept your capacity to make your own best choices. Focus on how to move forward with greater confidence instead of worrying about what you might have to give up in moving to the next level of living your purpose.

We all are endowed with a creative spark. Those who have recognized and cultivated this gift sleep soundly knowing their efforts will bear fruit. Time spent in non-creative activities is frustrating, leaving you worrying about the past and future. Having given up on the moment, there is nothing but mental dullness and anxiety. In this environment constant fear and doubt flourish like an opportunistic infection in an immuno-compromised individual. Now is the time to look back to past successes and rekindle the confidence and lightheartedness associated with mastery and success. You can do what you want knowing that the end result is not the goal but that living the creative life is the way. Trust in the grace that you are about to receive.

How can we re-educate ourselves and discover the creative spirit? Thich Nhat Hanh says the first step is to do nothing.[3] Stop trying to achieve because you believe that achievement leads to contentment. You can work hard all of your life, get yourself into a position where you could buy all of the things you thought would make you happy, and still end up feeling empty. You are not living from within if you find the actions and words of others bother or irritate you. At such times, you have given your power away and missed the point. On the other hand, if you know in your heart that you can be happy no matter what confronts you, then you have achieved all that you will ever need. Self confidence builds as you become more comfortable with your abilities to meet challenges. Correct inner self-talk can make things happen for you, but first you have to question yourself and honestly evaluate your current choice of words and feelings.

If you feel like a loser, you will lose. The lower you get, the more life will bring you down, but things will change once you discover that it is your attitude concerning your problems that controls everything. If you inwardly smile at misfortune and see it as a stepping stone, you are way ahead of the game. While others wail and moan over their challenges you overcome yours with confidence. It takes trust to tell yourself that you are confident when you do not feel that way. By telling yourself that you are part of the process, you allow yourself to move away from old labels such as "good" or "bad". When you drop judgment and trust the creative power within yourself, the brain makes new neuronal connections and you open the way for perfect self-expression.

How do you get to where you can live with ease and view your problems with a light heart? The first step is to make a commitment to yourself that the next time you find yourself lost in self pity, or upset over a situation, that you consciously make a decision to remain present and not allow yourself to get tied up in a frenzy of frustration or anger. By activating your patience you may find that this is not the time for the manifestation of your desire. Patience allows you to hold on to the knowledge that you can manifest that which you need and want. By focusing your dominant thoughts and behaviors on the positive, your quality of life and sense of satisfaction multiply. You eventually develop mastery in relation to the events in your life.

One way to go about bringing inner transformation with less of a jolt to your system, and in a less threatening way to your ego, is to begin to soften the words that you habitually use. Anthony Robbins in his bestselling book *Awaken the Giant Within: How to take immediate control of your mental, emotional, physical, & financial destiny*[4], lists many of the negative words we use. He tells readers to exchange them for words that express a more positive connotation. Instead of saying you are anxious, he recommends changing this expression to being "a little concerned," or "expectant." Instead of labeling yourself as being depressed, as 50 million Americans do, he explains that by using phrases such as "I am experiencing a calm before action," or "I am on the road to a turnaround," that the emotional intensity is softened by such a great extent, that instead of feeling upset or stuck over your situation, you recognize that your condition is simply a temporary state and you will successfully navigate your way to success.

When your thoughts are scattered your results will reflect this state of mind, but when you know exactly what you want, your thoughts and actions will lead you to where you need to be to make your dreams come true. As James Allen says in *As A Man Thinketh*, "Strong, pure, and happy thought build up the body in vigor and grace. The body is a delicate and plastic instrument, which responds readily to the thoughts by which it is impressed, and habits of thought will produce their own effects, good or bad, upon it."[5]

Some people are too intense. Like a laser, they bore through those around them, overpowering them with their energy. With piercing eyes, their intensity brings up images of The Inquisition. If you find yourself so intense that others want to move away from you, it is time to relax and gently focus on trust. Directing your mind to a place of belonging and connecting with others, where everyone wants the same things, will do much to soften your countenance. We all want to be happy, have enough money for the things we need and want, and feel like we fit in. If your energies of anger and judgment are palpable, your underlying emotion is fear. Such dense, dark energy is depressing (the calm before action?), and heavy. To extricate yourself from such binding energies, begin to practice patience by asking yourself what patience means to you.

You can begin your practice of expressing greater patience by jotting down your responses to the following questions:

1. What does it mean to be patient?
2. What virtues do you find associated with patience?
3. What ideas and beliefs do you have to let go of to become more patient?
4. When you review your answers to question # 3, what images of resistance come to mind?
5. What new idea or belief can you plant in your mind right now that will put you on the road to developing greater patience?

In moving toward your goals, if you over-expend your energies, you find yourself tense and tired all the time. Such intensity tends to keep people at arm's length and is draining. It takes so much energy to listen to someone who is not in contact with their own energy flow. Unfortunately, this is also true when it comes to hearing your own voice. Begin to quiet the commotion in your mind and start listening to the silence. Look for the space between your words. Rest in that space, welcome it and rejoice in the peace.

Whether we want to believe it or not, where we focus our thought is intimately associated with what we experience. In a relationship, if you choose to continually dwell on a conceived negative attribute of another, you will find what you are looking for. If you expect your spouse to react to a request or action in a certain way, you have effectively closed the door for them to act in any other way. That is unless the other person is consciously working on changing his or her conditioned responses.

Working on softening and making space for yourself and your relationships is hard work, as it takes repetition and trust to exercise your creative talents. Insights do not come as freebies. Inner work has to be done so that the conditioned mind no longer moves along the deep grooves of past experience. The conditions that allow for such work to proceed have to be desired and intentioned. One of the most common complaints I hear in my medical practice is, "I am tired of being tired." When you come to the place where you can truly say this, and are really searching for answers, more questions arise. Unfortunately too many people get overwhelmed at the enormity of the task and tell themselves there is no use in trying. They know it takes energy to focus but believe they are deficient in overall energy, when in reality they deplete their own energy in repetitive negative thoughts.

To become childlike again is to pay attention to where your predominant thoughts reside. At first you may think that all of this is just too much trouble, that you have no time for such contemplation, that you have no idea of which way to proceed, and that there is no reason to try to change your outlook or attitude, because you are who you are. Such beliefs keep you from moving ahead and douse any hope of finding peace. Think loosely, open your heart, and begin to experience compassion for yourself. You are worthy and deserving of it.

Self-fulfilling prophecy is a reality. Your thoughts make and maintain your reality. In computer jargon, a *Make* is a computer program used to automate the translation of one computer language into that of another so that the two can work interchangeably. The Make programs work by parsing, or breaking down, a language into characters that are meaningful to the other. A Make program also has to deal with a program's dependencies on other software or files.[21]

Make programs have limitations in that they have a lack of support for configuration-dependency management." This means that when there are changes in the system, Make does not know it needs to rebuild things. Many times when we are presented with change in our lives we become upset and the negative self-talk makes things harder than they are. We are dependent on the way things are and resist change. As noted in *Brainy Encyclopedia*[6], dependence in Behavioral Medicine is described as a continuum of physical and psychological attachments related to the concept of addiction—addiction being defined as uncontrollable compulsion to repeat a behavior regardless of it negative consequences.[7]

In the still popular book titled *Who Moved My Cheese? : An A-Mazing Way to Deal with Change in Your Work and in Your Life* by Spencer Johnson, M.D., the author uses the adventures, fears and courage of two mice and two "little people" to bring home the point that change is actually good and that it is not to be feared. When we continually focus on the way things have been, and desire for things to stay the way they are, we get stuck and eventually end up with no cheese. Haw, one of the "little people" began to change when he "learned to laugh at himself and at what he had been doing wrong."[8]

The problem here is that many of us find it almost impossible to laugh at ourselves or even joke about past difficult experiences. In our choice to persistently take life too seriously, the door to a more rewarding and pleasing life remains bolted. Seeing yourself in a new light and appreciating your past experiences, no matter how difficult they may have been, frees you from their grip.

When you can think this way you are able to drop old concepts and move on with a new appreciation of your experiences. Haw also did the following: "He reflected on the mistakes he had made in the past and used them to plan for his future. He had to admit that the biggest inhibitor to change lies with yourself, and that nothing gets better until *you* change."[9]

No one likes to focus on their problems and denial has a useful function in everyday life. Opportunity knocks when you start to realize that your life is not going the way you want it to go. You wake up one day and find the motivations that worked yesterday will no longer work for you today or tomorrow. All of a sudden everything becomes a chore. You begin to think that all that is asked of you has become a "pain in the neck," but have no idea why.

This is the time to focus on the problems and seek to determine their causes. You can still go about your daily routine, though you may find things do not bring you the same pleasure that they had in the past. As you focus on your problems, it is also important to ask your source, be it God, Buddha, or the Universe, for guidance. This is the time to listen intently and stay tuned in to clues that will help you navigate your way out of your current unpleasant condition. It is a time to activate your imagination and come up with solutions that will bring you satisfaction.

Simultaneously, as you seek answers to your dilemma, you are to affirm that the answers to your questions are manifesting for the good of all involved. This may include your family, friends, co-workers, or whomever is in your mind when you think about your issues. Work to look beyond your fears instead of focusing on them and project the best case scenario for others and yourself. Do what you have to and allow yourself to trust that things will work out to your satisfaction. Focus on the positive in everything and be thankful for all things even though you may be surrounded by negativity and difficult situations. This is a good time to look to the past and review how you came out of a bad situation by employing purposeful action. Take whatever small steps to which you are led, knowing that even the smallest action will start things moving in the desired direction. At this point do not forget the first step that was mentioned above which was to do nothing.

In the act of doing nothing, you allow yourself to work things out internally and play with possible outcomes based on choices that you have. Realize that the choices you have today will be different from the choices that you have tomorrow or next week. As you focus your attention on the best possible solution, more choices will become apparent to you. If you have been allowing another personality to stop you from moving in your own direction, it is time to recognize this and mentally release them. You were not put on this earth to please others; you were put here to express your own potential and give the world the gifts that only you have to offer. The toughest job for most is settling down enough and quieting the mind enough to discover what those gifts are.

If you get lost in the circular argument that you can never change things, just look to the science of neuronal plasticity. Scientists, specifically neurobiologists, can condition fear responses in their subjects. Our knowledge of the learning process has come a long way since Pavlov and his salivating dogs. Scientists can now tell us down to the molecular level how they believe associative learning occurs in the brain. Recent studies performed by Hugh T. Blair et al at New York University on fear conditioning have demonstrated that a neutral conditioned stimulus paired with an aversive unconditioned stimulus will lead to fear conditioning by association and co-stimulation of neural pathways. It has been known for some time that the lateral nucleus of the amygdala is the locus in the brain that controls the fear response. Through Blair's work, and the work of many others, it is has been shown that the movement of calcium across specific receptors (NMDA or N-methyl-D-aspartate receptors) in the brain mediates fear responses. When these receptors are occupied changes occur in the brain circuitry that supports short-term fear memory.

With an unconditioned fear response these same receptors and brain loci are stimulated to a greater degree. The higher intensity depolarization, or movement of calcium, sodium, and potassium along the axons, leading to the lateral nucleus of the amygdala causes signals to back-propagate into the dendrites (the part of the neuron that transports signals away from the source neuron). This colliding of impulses causes calcium to enter the neuron through different channels, referred to as "voltage-gated" calcium channels (VGCCs). Once both channels are activated and calcium is allowed to move through both the NMDA receptors and the VGCC's, this initiates the molecular cascade that produces long-term memory of the unconditioned response.[10]

No wonder it is so difficult to face your fears. The demons within are the result of intricate chemical processes of which the average person can neither see nor understand to their full extent. When these associations are made at a young age, the psyche keeps the original insult under raps and puts up defense mechanisms in its attempt to function optimally.

If we appreciate the mystery of what goes on in our minds and realize that scientists are still scratching the surface on how to put all of these facts together, it will serve us well to understand that what the mind can do, it can also undo. The point of focus here is exercising trust and knowing that the mind has the power to heal itself.

If this is the case, how do you get out of your mind's way to heal and remain healthy? Joel Goldsmith, in *The Art of Spiritual Healing,* stresses that if we can believe that there is no real or true disease and that the only reality is God or a higher power, then we can let go of illness and live healthy lives.[11] This may be hard to swallow, especially for someone who suffers from one of the many cancers known to human kind, or for those who have diabetes or cerebrovascular illnesses, such as strokes and heart disease, and whose lives are forever changed because of these diseases. On the other hand our current literature tells us that only 5% of cancers occur on a genetic basis while the other 95% are due to environmental causes: meaning lifestyle choices such as alcohol and tobacco abuse, over-eating, and sedentary lifestyles. How many people do you know who still smoke despite being aware that they are putting themselves at higher risk of lung cancer? Most explain their persistence in this vice with the comment, "Well, you have to die of something."

From this we can conclude that another point of focus is to take an active role in caring for your temple. That means going out of your way to do regular exercise, having enough discipline to avoid overeating, and being awake and aware enough not to use food as a sedative. Neuronal plasticity was a hot topic even twenty-five years ago when I was introduced to it as a psychobiology major. Though there is a much greater understanding of the molecular mechanisms involved in this plasticity, the bottom line for you is that the brain is indeed plastic, at least to a degree. When it comes to the mind and human spirit, it is true that nothing is written in stone. You can recondition even your most difficult to control behaviors and emotions, but you have to be willing to give up past grievances, slights, and abuses. You have to be willing to stand naked as you are, and bring the walls down that keep you from your true healthy self. The idea of blame has to be released. The ideal of health has to be addressed and supported with your every thought and action. You can do this, and it will only be as difficult as you believe it to be. If you believe that you have power in your life, and if you can accept the concept of grace, you will see change. Initially you may not know where help will come from, but as you focus on your health and the health of others, a teacher will come.

As this unfolds you will find yourself opening up to more people, you will be emotionally closer to your loved ones, and you will naturally spread good will and kindness to others as you accept kindness for yourself. All of this will take repetition and patience as your thoughts undo then restructure your interneuronal connections. New actions will follow new thoughts, so the sooner you start the sooner you find yourself feeling better. Focus on forgiveness as you gain a deeper appreciation for what you have had to do to survive. As you forgive others, your point of focus changes as you become grateful in everything. There are no right or wrong answers. There is just what you can offer in your transformation.

Focus on what you now have as if standing between two mirrors. If you have two eyes that see clearly, give thanks. If you have two arms, two legs, or even one leg and prosthesis, focus on what is going right in your life. Reclaim your power to choose for yourself those thoughts that will bring you higher. Abandon all thoughts of failure or unworthiness. You are here to make your contribution and blend with others in the mystery and mastery of life.

Notes: Point of Focus

1. Matthew Weschler, "How Lasers Work," See *Howstuffworks* at http://science.howstuffworks.com/laser.htm/printable.

2. Mihaly Csikszentmihalyi, *Flow: The Psychology of Optimal Experience* (New York: HarperCollins, 1990).

3. Thich Nhat Hanh, *Peace is Every Step: The Path of Mindfulness in Everyday Life*, (New York: Bantam Books, 1991), p.17.

4. Anthony Robbins, *Awaken the Giant Within: How to take control of your mental, emotional, physical, & financial destiny*, (New York, Fireside Books, Simon & Schuster, 1991), pp. 216-218.

5. James Allen, *As A Man Thinketh* (New York: Grosset & Dunlap), p. 34.

6. From: Brainy Encyclopedia, http://www.brainyencyclopedia/m/ma/make.html

7. Ibid.

8. Spencer Johnson, *Who Moved My Cheese? An A-Mazing Way to Deal with Change in Your Work and in Your Life*, (New York: G.P. Putnam's Sons, 1998), p. 70.

9. Ibid, p. 71.

10. Hugh T. Blair, et al, "Synaptic Plasticity in the Lateral Amygdala: A Cellular Hypothesis of Fear Conditioning," *Learning and Memory* 8:pp.229-242, 2001.

11. Joel S. Goldsmith, *The Art of Spiritual Healing*, (New York; Harper & Row, 1959), pp. 73-81.

CHAPTER 3

Praise Your Perfection

The power of praise is often overlooked as a method of getting the best from yourself and others. Children who grow up continually criticized will, once they become parents, unintentionally criticize their offspring. It is what they have learned and unless they have a desire to relearn a better way, they will pass this behavior on to their offspring ad infinitum. On the other hand authentic praise empowers the recipient. When was the last time you remember being pleased by someone's performance at a stage play or a concert? Did you reach out and tell them that their performance impressed you enough to momentarily drop your own concerns and worries, and that you were inspired? You do not have to be at a play to witness an act of kindness, an encouraging statement at a meeting, or a friendly smile, but wherever you are, you can take note. See how long you can carry the impression with you, and how it changes the way you interact with others for the remainder of the day.

As you can see, this is not the kind of praise given to a higher power for the gift of Grace. This is giving attention and recognition to another human being because you appreciate their value. Some will minimize this action by thinking it is simply passing out "warm fuzzies," but at the basic level, people thrive on appreciation and encouragement. Just the other day a patient's husband remarked that if we knew all that a mother did in a day, between getting the children ready for school, preparing meals, acting as chauffeur, planning social events, and taking care of a spouse as well as herself, a man would be surprised and even shocked. He would definitely be more appreciative. This gentleman has watched his wife slowly wither away from the effects of breast cancer that has spread to the lining of her lungs and her brain. Though she currently has no evidence of residual cancer she continues to decline from the long term side effects of her therapy. As she slows down, his work increases, but he is more than happy to do all that he can for her because 1) he loves her very much and 2) he appreciates all that she did for him and the family in her healthy years.

Through his recognition of her contributions, he is now able to appreciate in himself his ability and willingness to lovingly care for her. It is not that he is telling himself that he is any better than anyone else in caring for her. Instead he can see that he is a better person through his unconditional giving to the woman who had given so much of herself when he and his family were in need. Her misfortune with the cancer has given him a chance to see more clearly a loving and caring side of himself.

No two accomplishments are of equal value as no two individuals possess the same abilities. A healthy personal yardstick is based on past performance, and is not shaded by the opinion of anyone else. It is ok to build yourself up and it is not an ego trip when giving to another is done mindfully and unselfishly. It is healthy and rewarding to give in this way and it is acceptable to take credit for it. In the realm of Buddhists you are working off bad karma. For Christians one may be atoning for past sins. In any religion, doing selflessly for another is a reason to feel good and indeed feeling good may be the result of doing for others. With all of the challenges and expectations we face it is this little extra positive reinforcement that many times can help get us through a difficult trial.

There is a word, *doxophobia,* with which you may not be familiar, unless you happen to be a psychology major, clinical psychologist, or a psychiatrist. To be *doxophobic* means to possess an abnormal and persistent fear of expressing opinion or of receiving praise. Individuals who suffer from this fear have failed to continually reset their compasses in relation to their own changing needs. Instead of plotting their own courses, they were as described by Warren Bennis in *On Becoming A Leader,*[1] as overly influenced by their elders or peers. They failed to invent themselves for themselves and have fallen into the "dark side" of Eric Eriksson's Eight Stages of Development. They learned basic mistrust instead of trust, shame and doubt instead of autonomy, guilt instead of initiative, inferiority instead of industry, identity confusion instead of identity, and isolation instead of intimacy.

These first six stages of Eriksson's theory cover an individual up to the age of forty.[2] The seventh stage refers to stagnation instead of generativity that occurs from age 40 to 60. During this time one who is generous will teach the younger generation useful concepts they have learned throughout their life. From the age of sixty to death the issues of integrity versus despair are dealt with as this is the time to contemplate decisions as to whether your life was a success or failure.

There is always a choice as to where you decide to place your attention. A healthy choice is to appreciate your every action whether you thought it was right or wrong at the time. Many times decisions have to be made with an inadequate amount of information. With introspection and retrospection, you find there are no real mistakes. Every choice made contributed to adaptation, growth, and maturity. To choose judgment and self-criticism is to miss the point, since to know what works you have to know what doesn't work. William Martin tells us this beautifully in *The Parent's Tao Te Ching,* with his story entitled "Opposites Are Necessary:"

Opposites Are Necessary

"If you want your children to be generous,
You must first allow them to be selfish.
If you want them to be disciplined,
You must first allow them to be spontaneous.
If you want them to be hard-working,
You must first allow them to be lazy.
This is a subtle distinction,
And hard to explain to those who criticize you.
A quality cannot be fully learned
Without understanding its opposite."[3]

Praise functions as a means to connect with another person, especially one whom you are teaching or working with. Work and instruction move along smoothly when there are positive words and shared feelings. A child will blossom and excel when given authentic praise. In order to give praise you have to feel good about yourself. When you have the self-esteem to praise your own efforts, your progress in whatever endeavor you choose also benefits in a linear fashion, instead of chopping along with one step forward then two steps back. The internal positive feedback acts as a stimulus for one small success after another.

What happens if you dislike yourself or even worse, hate yourself? How in the world can you give others true praise and recognition if you believe you are broken or inadequate? The amount of work required to overcome these tendencies is overwhelming and intimidating. Perhaps you have a few self-help and positive-thinking books on your bookshelves. To date, they have not worked as you wished they would, so you believe you're stuck and have to live out the rest of your life in mediocrity. If the internal battle of good over evil escalates, you may find yourself tired and near exhaustion. This negative loop can perpetuate itself unless you take action to alter it.

If you struggle to remove yourself from feelings of worthlessness and shame, working hard to prove your goodness, the result may be that there is nothing left at the end of the day to enjoy. Too critical to ever pat yourself on the back, you may push yourself until you can't go any more. This creates fertile ground for anger because of exhaustion and the unmet need for rest. What is it that you are looking for? Are you seeking an end to your problems and needs? Are you looking for Shangri-La? If you figuratively find yourself in the slums, it may be because your thoughts dwell on your deficiencies and not your strengths.

Such belief systems do not go down easily. You think you have to keep making changes to improve yourself so that you can control your anger, manage your temper, and exercise your patience. All of that energy is turned back on itself without a productive direction. It has nowhere to go so it keeps you in your mire. As Cheri Huber tells us in *Regardless of What You Were Taught to Believe: There is Nothing Wrong With You,* "Self-hate is terrified that you will make being kind to yourself a habit."[4] Once you make the decision to take care of yourself and treat yourself well, all of the stops are pulled and the negative self-talk escalates itself like a solar flare of the sun. Its goal is to stir up more fear; your job is to see the fear and say, "so what?"

Cheri Huber also tells us what we think we already know, and that is: "We must become our own best friend. We must learn to give to ourselves and to receive from ourselves unconditional love and acceptance."[5] Everyone has experienced trauma and shame in their lifetime. The way we deal with these experiences determines how comfortable we are in our day-to-day, person-to-person encounters. Defense mechanisms are developed to protect the ego from painful or shameful events. A number of common clinical syndromes are now viewed as the result of chronic dissociation (a lack of connection in one's thoughts, memories, feelings, actions or sense of identity). These include eating disorders, depression, obsessive compulsive disorder, phobias, and panic disorder. Multiple personality disorder, which is now called dissociative identity disorder by the American Psychiatric Association, is the extreme result of chronic dissociation.[6]

The one thing that people can agree upon is that life is a paradox. The struggles and pain, the ups and downs, the sadness and the joy, for the lucky ones, are in balance. For some it seems they receive the lion's share of misery. To ask one to praise their perfection when all they have in front of them is one struggle after another, one disappointment followed closely by the next, makes you wonder how they ever go on. Thomas Moore, in *The Soul's Religion* tells us that, in a way, these individuals are also expressing their own perfection. He reminds us of the following: "We become most who we are when we allow the spirit to dismember us, unsettling our plans and understandings, remaking us from the very foundations of our existence."[7] He is telling us that when our lives are falling apart, we are most closely touching life. This is nothing of which to be shameful or fearful.

The pervading message is this: No matter what you are going through or how long you think you have to work to survive and expend effort to figure things out, when you allow whatever is happening to you to just happen without fighting or resisting, then you are living in reality. Suffering is minimized by not wanting things to be a certain way. Maybe that is why the Burger King commercial is so appealing when they tell you that you can "Have It Your Way." Where else in life can you always have things your way? You will not find such conditions at work, home, or even on vacation, as there will always be something pulling at you from one direction or another.

What if you made the choice to label every situation that you have experienced as being perfect? Look at the pressure that would take off of you. Feel the relief that comes when you don't critique your every action or your every choice. This is not to advocate that you drop all responsibility, but if you just gave up the need for blame and the need to have things be just so all of the time, then you could simply relax in your own perfection. No need to keep the inner judge employed. You could lay off the super ego and begin to examine the roles of some of your sub-personalities. It makes for interesting examination and is enlightening.

In spiritual psychology a sub-personality is one of the many inner "players" or actors within your mind. Each one expresses an attitude or belief that you have, yet they are not to be labeled as being good or bad. When one sub-personality dominates your life you feel out of control. When you take the time to identify and recognize some of these actors, your awareness into your motivation increases and you develop the ability to integrate these sub-personalities. Once you accept the critic within, you take away its power to rule you and make you feel uncomfortable. You may still listen to him but you will do so as an observer and not as the victim. When you begin to praise each one of these inner parts of yourself for how well they play their roles and how perfect their interactions are, they will open up to you and you will feel less divided. The initial step is to get over the idea that there is something wrong with you when you begin to first identify these entities.

We are more than our personalities and their constituents. Our earthly bodies are engineering wonders of their own. On the one side they are so delicate and intricate, functioning within tight parameters such as the acid-base balance or the pH of the blood. The range that is conducive to good health does not allow for much variation and has a span of 7.35-7.45. To experience even less than a one point change in either direction leaves life hanging in the balance. Those individuals living with insulin-dependent diabetes who have experienced a diabetic coma, or in medical lingo what is referred to as diabetic ketoacidosis, know just how ill such a minor change in body chemistry can make them.

The fact that we as a species have been given the talent and intelligence to learn about the physiology of the body, and then take steps to correct it, says a great deal for the power of the mind. The body's ability to repair itself after a number of unwelcomed insults is also a reason for praise. In the practice of oncology as well as the other branches of medicine, we have all seen individuals - some on death's door - recover a degree of health. Every oncologist has a handful of patients whom they know should not still be here because their diseases had been so advanced that the odds of successful treatment were close to zero. The bizarre thing is that many of these patients never know how fortunate they are until someone tells them. Their return to health is taken for granted.

Yesterday, on a six month followup, I had the pleasure of seeing a long-term breast cancer survivor. Eight years ago while being treated with chemotherapy, she developed metastatic disease to the brain. She was referred to a nearby university for gamma-knife radiation therapy. Her tumor shrunk and she has remained in remission with an excellent quality of life. She is free of any of the toxic effects of whole- brain radiation that we see in those fortunate to live beyond two years. Her mentation and physical function are normal. She has an excellent memory and lives a life as if she had never been afflicted with cancer. She had no idea that she was a walking miracle. She seemed ready to hear this and was matter of fact about her continued gift of life as she affirmed that God had taken care of her.

The natural ability our bodies have to maintain the flow of blood through our arteries and veins is itself a wondrous work of art. Man is not capable of developing such a system of intertwining cascades that function so perfectly on a consistent basis. When you receive a cut or an injury, unless you are a Hemophiliac or suffer from one of the very rare platelet disorders, you take it for granted that your blood is going to clot. You are so sure of it that minor cuts or bruises are only an inconvenience.

You do not see the automatic, instantaneous biochemical events occurring within the body as the intrinsic and extrinsic coagulation systems go into action. Inert chemical precursors are converted into active compounds by co-factors such as calcium, and blood-clotting Factor VII, and Factor VIII. The body's coagulation system is dependent on the normal functioning of the liver. The liver is the source of important clotting glycoproteins, such as fibrinogen.

Once there is a cut, at the end of the coagulation cascade, fibrinogen is converted into fibrin. At this point the meshwork has been created to act as a breeding point for clot formation. As platelets, which are flowing in the blood, crash into this mesh a clot is formed and you stop bleeding. If anything, we should praise the intricacies and wisdom of our bodies that keep us healthy and alive.

False praise does not help anyone. Most individuals, no matter what age, can differentiate between what is really said and what is expressed. The true meaning comes across only when we are sincere in expressing words of encouragement. It means more when you stop what you are doing, look the individual in the eyes and tell them how you appreciated their contribution or action. It doesn't mean as much if you give a cursory "nice job," while you are frantically walking past to get to your destination on time. When the message comes from the heart both the giver and receiver feel the connection.

When you give praise to another you demonstrate to them that you care about how they are doing. This is especially so when the receiver is working at a new task or learning a new skill. Too many times the learner is faced with one frustration after another and begins to feel overwhelmed. Without encouragement they may come to the point where they tell themselves they are wasting their time trying to master the task or subject. While moving along the steep slope of the learning curve, the difference between success and failure can depend on the type of praise one receives.

For someone skilled in the gift of moderation for self-praise, we can appreciate their position in having been fortunate to have had others give them authentic praise along their way. For them, internal self-talk is comforting and assuring. It keeps them on the task at hand. Praise does not cost anything, but it does take the effort of one person caring for another. If you are truly pleased with the progress of another, in no way will you be accused of giving false praise. Parents wonder if too much praise will make a child overconfident and foster a false sense of mastery. Any child who has been encouraged to think for himself knows what is true and what is not true. Just because a child is younger in years doesn't mean that they are unaware of their own inner wisdom. An astute child will call your bluff and put you back in your place as if doing you a favor when they catch you passing out false praise.

Before giving praise, be sure you are satisfied with that to which you are responding. Don't just praise someone to hear your own voice. True praise is the expression of genuine caring, surprise, or amazement. The tone of the voice, the body language, and the look in your eyes convey the truth of what you are saying.

For the next week look to see how often you offer praise to another and rate the sincerity of what you are saying. See if you can bring your sincerity rating higher as the week goes on. Also, when you feel that you have been doing a job worthy of praise and no praise is forthcoming, offer yourself your own praise. Remember that little child inside is always there even though you have tuned out his or her voice over the years. We are all worthy of praise. Too many young people end up in trouble because of the unrelenting criticism they receive. You can tell the criticism has hit the mark when you hear them criticize a friend for a mistake, or when they call themselves stupid when they can't figure out a math problem for homework.

In order to keep your children looking up to you every time you call their name, it is necessary to sometimes pleasantly ask how they are doing. There should be no agenda concerning your wanting something from them. It is healthy for them to often hear how you appreciate them simply for who they are. Offering a few simple words of praise will give you a special place in their lives. The best way to improve your standing in any group, be it a family or a business organization, is to give out genuine heartfelt praise freely.

Don't worry about giving others too much of a big head or about making them feel better about themselves. As those around you get more comfortable in their roles, so will your life and experiences be more comfortable and rewarding. These things are so simple but too many people worry about giving their praise in fear that others will develop a superiority complex. Even if they did, it would be much less harmful to them than an inferiority complex. A word of praise can keep someone on track as they learn to master a particular discipline or action. On the other hand, a word of harsh or unthoughtful criticism can freeze someone in their tracks. When this happens, nobody wins.

You can look at giving your praise to others as a contribution to their welfare. You are helping them build a healthy sense of self-worth. It is an opportunity to do something great without actually having to do anything other than using you words, feelings, and authenticity. Praise will give its recipient a reason to smile, and that smile reflected back to you will warm your heart. Through your effort you are both ushered into the moment.

It is so easy to strike out and blame yourself or others when things appear to go wrong. This action becomes an easy way out of taking responsibility for what has happened. With some concentrated effort, it is possible to interject words of praise and encouragement even in the face of adversity. Begin to look at all situations you face as *necessary*. You are unconsciously absorbing information that will become useful at a later time. It may be a small insight but that seed, once planted, will make itself visible in its own time. Be patient with yourself. Get away from critical self-talk and replace it with the soothing balm of praise for who you are right now.

Notes: The Praise of Perfection

1. Warren Bennis, *On Becoming A Leader* (Cambridge, MA: Perseus Books, 1994), p. 62.

2. http://www.ship.edu/~cgboeree/erikson.html Eric Erikson was a Freudian ego-psychologist who developed a theory of identity development expanding on Freud's theory of stages. Erikson noted that development proceeds by the epigenetic principle in that we develop through a predetermined unfolding of our personalities in eight stages. Progress through each stage depends on the success of the previous stages.

3. William Martin, *The Parent's Tao Te Ching: A New Interpretation* (New York: Marlowe & Company, 1999), p. 61.

4. Cheri Huber, *Regardless of What You Were Taught To Believe...There is Nothing Wrong With You* (Keep It Simple Books, 2001), pp.104-105.

5. Ibid, p. 86.

6. Maggie Phillips & Claire Frederick, *Healing the Divided Self*, cited from http://users.lmi.net/mphillips/chapter1.html.

7. Thomas Moore, *The Soul's Religion: Cultivating a Profoundly Spiritual Way of Life* (New York, 2002), p. 89.

CHAPTER 4

Conditions We Live By

In trying to live up to self-imposed conditions, or conditions others attempt to place on us, we set our own boundaries. Such boundaries are sometimes difficult to define, especially those surrounding close contacts like family members. If we are in a less than optimal position concerning boundaries because of unconscious conditioning, we become our own jailers. With self-reflection it is possible to decipher which conditions foster approval, and which bring disapproval from significant others as well as work associates.

Some parents set up boundaries by withholding affection until their expectations are met. If a room is not tidied up, or a request not carried out, defenses are put in motion and assumptions are made that "my children don't listen." Irrespective of the current perspective of the child, some parents will interrupt what the child is doing and proceed to make demands. Many parents tend to forget the preoccupations of childhood and are quick to label the child as lazy or disobedient. This kind of labeling can lead to self-fulfilling prophecies which act to the detriment of the child. A common, corrective parental measure is negative reinforcement, or taking something pleasurable away from the delinquent child such as television or computer time.

When pushed to seek other forms of punishment, parents may threaten and yell, believing that unless they raise their voice, they will not be heard. Thus begins a lifelong dance of disruption. No wonder so many children tune things out.

All things in life are based on conditions. We like to think that we do things for legitimate and practical reasons, but in fact, much of our daily lives are spent in behaviors based on past conditioning. We go to work on the condition that we will receive a paycheck for the work we have performed. This may be the case even though the work does not feed our soul, or it leaves us feeling empty at the end of the day. We are polite so that others will view us in good standing. We give of our time and energies so that when we are in need, hopefully someone will be there for us, believing in and living by the Golden Rule. No matter how enlightened we think we are, it is human to be shaped by the conditions that surround us.

As we walk further on the path to enlightenment, with intention and right effort, we may be able to look back and realize some of the conditions to which we have allowed ourselves to adhere. At this point we can make a conscious decision to move in the direction of mindful and intentional action. But alas, we are merely human and no matter how hard we try, we are not capable of living mindfully all of the time. Mindfulness can remain our goal, and with practice, we will experience more and more moments of being present. In doing so we weaken the conditions of the past that served to keep us stuck.

When conditions become overwhelming and approach the breaking point, we may forget to do things from the heart. If external forces become our primary motivators we end up doing things because we feel that we have to. With no time allotted to contemplate what our real needs are, we keep chasing the carrot only to find that once we bite into it, there is a bigger, brighter carrot around the next corner. Thus the cycle perpetuates itself. We end up going around in circles and finally give up only when exhaustion sets in and we are without any reserve energy or strength. Then the feeling of being stuck sets in and the sense of despair predominates in our minds.

How do we move away from external sources of motivation and stop chasing rewards for what we do? There are ways to get into the flow of performing a task, getting deeply involved with the task, and feeling our own presence with such involvement. Mihaly Csikzentmihalyi explains *Flow* as "the state in which people are so involved in an activity that nothing else seems to matter."[1] He tells us that the individuals who are in touch with their own experience, whether viewed as good or bad, are the ones who find themselves the happiest. If you discover an activity that you love more than anything else in the world, you become so engrossed in the task at hand that the activity itself becomes its own reward. The ability to drop the need for a reward will express itself once you start doing the thing that you love the most.

Many parents today use rewards to get their children to do what they want them to do. Such methods will never consistently be effective since the motivation to perform is external to the child and does not come from within.

There are even health-related websites that reward children for eating right and exercising. No wonder we keep running after the prize since it has been held out in front of us since our earliest memories.

There is so much "if/then" mentality today that it takes us away from appreciating the mysterious and unknown components of everyday life. Many of us have lost the capacity to enjoy spontaneity. Afraid of taking risks, we chase the "sure thing" instead. The vast majority of us have become people who are terrified of uncertainty. We want to be guaranteed in every aspect of life, and for some that includes a guarantee that cancer chemotherapy will work. It is as if we are we are existing under the delusion that we were meant to live forever. Where did we ever get such a wild idea? Are we so frail and weak as a population that we have to deny that our lives are limited? The unknown has that kind of effect on us. It is time to awaken to the condition and the reality that our bodies have been designed for planned obsolescence. Only then can we truly live.

Everything in life is based on conditions. If you don't get enough sleep at night you will not function effectively the following day. If you treat others cruelly you will have no friends and many enemies. Forcing yourself to do things that you do not truly love will leave you exhausted and bitter. With all these conditions surrounding everything we do, the central question becomes: How do we make conditions right to produce the fruits that will make us happy?

Right off the bat, the one key concept to grasp is that "things or stuff" will not bring happiness. Work as hard as you want, buy everything that you think will make you happy, and you will find that you are still wanting. That new sports car will one day get scratched, the boat's bright, shiny and new hull will fade in the sun and salt water, and the new television or computer will be outdated in a year or two. In the conversations between His Holiness the Dalai Lama and Howard Cutler in *The Art of Happiness at Work*,[2] they discuss the development of self-understanding as a way to find greater happiness. It has more to do with having the skill to perform a particular type of job. The self-understanding they are talking about is based on the recognition of your own strengths, and realizing that you can generate your own happiness by living out the virtues that you naturally express without effort.

We have all met individuals who are innately kind. Their every word and action exudes kindness. They treat all persons the same regardless of social status. They are just as content saying hello to the office maintenance engineer as they are greeting the CEO. They, on a practical and functional level, see everyone as equal. Their expressions of giving are authentic and most times not even recognizable to them. Only when it is brought to their attention by a sincere "thank you," do they stop to take note of the root of their actions. Even so, they respond by saying the reason they are here is to be kind, or that it is the way that they would want to be treated.

We like to think that we do things for legitimate and practical reasons, but much of the day's activities are performed from the roots of past conditioning. We go to work and get a paycheck to maintain a certain standard of living. How many of us do our work and believe that it is part of our calling. In *A New Breed of Work Force Demands a New Breed of Manager*, Tom Brown sites the work of Martha Finney, who sought the reasons some individuals found joy in their work. She found that those having a joyful attitude toward work held onto their personal values. They knew what they enjoyed doing and they sought jobs which met that need. They remained optimistic even in the face of adversity, even when their struggles concerned moving along other career paths. These individuals also felt that their work was that of their calling.

How do we line up our inner world with the outer when it comes to the conditions that we face on the job? If you believe that you are stuck in a job where your talents are not being fully expressed, what steps can you take to begin to transition into a position where you are able to give your best and feel that you are growing and learning everyday? It does no good to blame yourself for the position that you are in. In the past you may have been completely satisfied with your job situation, but over time you may have grown out of the position. Now you seek greater challenges and possibly desire a complete change. Taking time to reflect on the concrete things that you did in the past that gave you satisfaction will help you frame your future. Listing the experiences where you found yourself in a state of flow and reliving those moments in quiet contemplation will help rekindle those feelings. When you begin to get a hint of the direction in which you wish to proceed, then immerse yourself in that activity or subject, but do not force yourself in any way. You have planted the seed and now you have to nurture it. Keep things simple and daily ask yourself: What is the next step that I have to take to make this change a reality?

The task is to look for the conditions you hold up for yourself that keep you in your own, limited sphere of thinking. What do you tell yourself every moment, on a day-to-day basis, that inhibits you from looking at your life in a way that keeps you from balance? With which aspect/s of your life do you find yourself struggling? It may be that you are grappling with a work issue or a family issue. Your challenge may be financial or related to family health issues. It may be related to a chronic pain that you have been experiencing. Whatever it is, there are conditions that keep you unaware.

It is not unusual to experience anxiety when you begin to explore the tough issues we are talking about. You are mustering the courage to chip away at old beliefs that have kept you in your limited and restricted state. These beliefs had you working much harder than necessary, simply because you assumed that, in order to get the job done, you needed to expend a great deal of effort. This is not the time to beat yourself up, but it is the time to begin to take care of yourself.

How do you take care of yourself when your past conditioning has told you that you have to always keep pushing and never let up? Now that your nervous system is so revved up, it has forgotten how to relax. Friends and family tell you to loosen up but you don't know how. You are living under the belief that unless you continually strive, you will never achieve anything of value. The problem becomes that, in such a state, you are incapable of appreciating all of the good that you now have. You don't plant a seed in the ground expecting corn to grow and dig it back up every day to check on its progress. You plant the seed, water it and on occasion remove surrounding weeds, then you let nature do the rest.

The first step in moving yourself to a place where you can have a chance to relax is to allow yourself to slow down. You have to convince yourself that it is safe to take it easy for a time. It is time to regroup—a time to reassess your priorities and develop a new paradigm concerning what you expect out of the gift of your life. In order to slow yourself down, you first have to be willing to remain open to all of the fears that you have carried along with you. This is far from easy. It may be the most difficult thing that you ever do. You have to place a bridle on your mind, then gently send it a new message that things are not the way you always thought they were.

It is time to admit to yourself, without blame, that you were wrong. It can be done with gentleness and compassion if you allow yourself the privilege of loving kindness. You have to convince your mind that it can stop living out of fear and begin living in an attitude of trust. In the places where you tell yourself no, you must entertain the notion that just maybe some of the goals that you see for yourself are indeed possible. These goals, however, are internally based and may include the goal to begin to see your life as it really is. It is as if you have to become a salesman for your imagination: go back in memory, find the root of each and every fear, and pull them out one at a time with the clear voice of reason. Let that voice be one of a trusted adult, wise with experience, as it speaks to your lost child. Slowly you will make the shift from a fear-based imagination to a healthy, positive-based one.

Part of the unwrapping of past conditions involves a need to drop all blame for the reasons why you believe things are the way they are today. If you have been telling yourself that your past family situation has held you back, or that you missed out on a quality education, you need to let go of these thoughts. Past financial concerns have to be put behind and a realistic assessment of your current condition and potential need to be reviewed. If you blame a parent for you current situation, you must begin to forgive them.

Usually, the first step in forgiveness is making the rationalization that those to be forgiven did the best that they could. Most of us do the best that we can in all situations. Such messages to the self are understood only on the intellectual level. Getting to the heart of forgiveness requires us to view our parents in a sea of compassion. It helps to realize that if we were in their exact situation we would have reacted in much the same way. We all come along with a great deal of baggage including all of the unfinished business relating to our parents. Our choices are to continue blaming them for all of our problems or to accept our own responsibility and pick up where they left off. In doing the latter we free ourselves and our children of the conditions of the past.

Softening the heart takes time. It usually doesn't happen overnight, but it can be equated to a tug-of-war, where one day you are more accepting and understanding, and the next day you have no patience whatsoever. So be it; tomorrow is another day. With time you will notice an overall softening, but it takes more patience than you think you possess. Here is where trust and grace come into play. You have to trust that you will find unconditional peace.

To relax the mind you have to allow yourself to relax your muscles. When you know that you are holding on somewhere in your body, be it your neck or back or jaw, it is possible to use that tension in a way that you can instruct your mind to relax around that tension. Instead of letting the mind do what it wants to do about this tension, which is to whirlwind around it and tense up further, it is in your power to instruct the mind to chill and just observe. It is like the inner critic of a writer during the writing of a first draft. Here the critic needs to take a vacation and ship off on a trip to one of the Hawaiian Islands. It needs to be assured that you will call it back for its expertise when you begin the second draft where the critic's work is essential.

What conditions do you hold for yourself that may be keeping you back? Maybe you are so wrapped up in receiving approval that everything you do is rooted in pleasing others. At work, you may be expected to work longer hours than you had originally planned for, but in order to keep peace and feel like you fit in, you work beyond your limits. You keep your thoughts to yourself, and when the inner tension builds, you can't figure out why. Continuing along this track allows anger to build, which is manifested as irritability.

Who are you trying to please with your behavior? Is there a specific person whose approval you are trying to win? They will come to mind when you start pushing yourself beyond what you feel is healthy. When you recognize this it is a perfect opportunity to ask yourself why you feel it is necessary to please them. What authority figures from your past are they a substitution for? Once you discover the hidden connection, it is time to ask yourself what it is that you really want to do. You must make a commitment to sort out all of the jumbled and mixed messages you have been giving yourself. Because of your dependency and fear you chose not to listen to your own voice. The price has been that you have never given yourself a chance to get to know who you really are. You surrendered your right to get to like yourself, and now as you are ready to take responsibility, you find there are a number of things about yourself that you really dislike. It is a difficult and awkward place to be. It is a place where no one would want to take your place, and no one can. You have to go it alone and sometimes it is only this incredible feeling of discomfort that will move you forward.

How many times have you thought or said, "I'll be happy when....?" Many of us falsely believe that when we make a predetermined amount of money that all of our troubles will miraculously vanish and we will be forever happy. This is our shot at security and a grappling with control. Unfortunately it just doesn't work that way. Others feel that once the children are grown and through school then they'll be free to live their own lives unimpeded. Still, others think that once they retire they will be liberated from the wheel of work and life will be good. Freed from tolerating the quirks of others, their energies can be directed toward doing the things that truly feed them. It is so important to look ahead with mindfulness so that when the days mentioned above do come about, we won't awaken to the surprise that life is not what we expected.

Happiness in life is also based on certain conditions. These are not difficult concepts to grasp; in fact they may be so simple that many disregard them because of their simplicity. As Mary Kay Mueller tells us in *Taking Care of Me: The Habits of Happiness*[4], there are twelve habits of happiness that we need to be mindful of. They are listed below.

Ask for what you want	Gratitude and giving
Being here now	Hugs and touch
Change your self talk	Insulate against negativity
Dream and set goals	Journal
Expecting the best	Keep on keeping on
Feel all your feelings	Lighten up and laugh

In the recommendation concerning **asking for what you want**, we might initially believe that we are quite comfortable with this concept. In viewing the results we obtain from our requests, however, it is often easy to see that something has gone wrong. No one really wants bad things to happen, but by disregarding our own wishes and not adhering to the concept of "right thought/right word," it is no wonder that unfortunate events do happen. We see the success of another and in a moment of weakness, instead of sharing in their joy, we find ourselves jealous. This is poison to the mind and brings unhappiness our way. Sure, we all know this on the intellectual level, but in order to live to our full potential it is time to pay attention to every word and thought and ask for that which is beneficial to all parties.

In asking for what you want, it is helpful to remember the adage that the "squeaky wheel" gets the grease. It is not that you have to make a pest of yourself, but you do have to make your needs known. This may be difficult for those who have come along in life by way of neglecting their own needs because of playing the role of peacekeeper in a family. If as a child your needs were ignored, you were effectively taught that what you wanted and needed was not important. It takes great effort to undo such damage, but unless the challenge to change is undertaken, you will continue to go along in life having difficulty meeting even your basic needs. At every chance you get, practice asking for what you want.

When it comes to **being here now,** we all know that this is something to always strive for, but if that is the case then why don't we practice more of it and stay alert as to when our buttons are being pushed. Stimulus-response action can be a lifesaver in a dangerous situation, such as reflexively slamming on the brakes when your subconscious tells you that someone is running a traffic light. On the other hand, if you persistently react with anger over otherwise petty comments directed toward you, then there is work to be done.

Eckhart Tolle, in *The Power of Now: A Guide to Spiritual Enlightenment*[5], tells us that an easy and direct way to become present is to listen to the silence. This not only pertains to getting quiet in meditation, but also in the arena of everyday activities. We can listen to all of the noise around us and still tune into the underlying silence. In our conversations we can become aware of the silence in between the words that we and others speak. The space between each of our in-breaths and out-breaths is loaded with silence. He explains that, in being present, we have chosen to allow our inner observer to do just that, and in doing so we take our attention away from physical and mental forms, thus making way for pure consciousness or presence. This is a practice that can be developed by anyone and has been part of the expansion of consciousness by the human race even before the inception of recorded time.

In discussing the next heading, **change your self-talk,** Anthony Robbins does all of the work for us in *"Awakening the Giant Within."*[6] He lists mediocre words that we commonly use and gives suggestions for the use of more powerful, dynamic, to the point, and expressive ones. His tack is that by using high energy words we facilitate the creation of that which we seek. Those going around all day telling themselves that they can't perform a specific task or begin to take steps toward a particular goal and then give up, seem to be saying more than anything, that they simply do not want to do anything to achieve satisfaction, acceptance, or balance.

Experiment for yourself. The next time you discover your frustration levels rise, ask yourself what it is you are telling yourself in the current situation. Each time, you will find that your self-talk is bringing you back to a past frustration that you were unable to resolve. When you have the courage to listen to exactly what you are saying, slowing down to see the images in your mind that your words produce, you have given yourself the power to forever change the way you will react to recurrent frustrations. Remind yourself often during this exercise of the following: that was then, this is now. The words are simple to say. The hard part is being disciplined enough to stay with what comes up and not judge yourself or allow yourself to fall back into your old habits.

The next section, **dream and set goals,** is your chance to have some fun. In this category there is no reason to limit yourself to what you presently feel might be realistic for you. The important thing to realize is that even though you are going to allow yourself to dream big, that when you move to make your dreams a reality, you do so in small steps. The way to your mark can be achieved by setting and meeting a number of short-term, doable goals, instead of trying to bite off a big chunk all at once. When we intend to read Dostoyevsky's *The Idiot,* it is useless to try to achieve that goal in one setting. Such an undertaking can be achieved if you use the Evelyn Woods speed-reading method, but that would severely detract from the pleasure of taking your time to savor each character's unique personality.

It helps to remember that when setting new goals, it is not the attainment of the goal itself that brings satisfaction. It is the day-to-day activities bringing challenges, enjoyment, and growth that are the means in setting conditions so that you may experience the state of flow with greater frequency. Taking the first step and then each successive step that you are led to take is the way to making your dreams a reality.

When it comes to **expecting the best,** there may be issues concerning your worthiness to receive the best that there is. If your conditioning has you accepting anything less than the best it is time to get to work on your self-talk and get busy doing some reprogramming. It is easy to look at what others have achieved and in comparing yourself to their accomplishment, find yourself lacking. The idea is not to compare yourself to any other individual. It is much more useful to compare how you operate on a day-to-day basis now compared to how you have done so in the past. A useful question to ask is: do I feel more comfortable in my skin today than I did yesterday? Realize that in every endeavor that you undertake that you are indeed doing your best and you will receive the necessary best that will fill your need at the moment.

As you **feel your feelings,** it is necessary to realize that if you have lived in a state of denial all of your life, you will not exactly know what it is you are feeling at any particular time. Your thoughts may be cloudy, the feelings you experience may be mixed or ambivalent, or you may simply be numb from all of the years of living in a self-protective mode. In a sense, what you have to do is thaw, both mentally and physically. The thawing process can be very frustrating unless you practice patience at the same time. As you begin this process and allow yourself to feel, one of the first feelings to surface will be anger.

Anger in itself is not a good or bad emotion. It can be very useful to you when used in the proper way. Anger is full of energy. Instead of turning that anger inward and ending up with chronic depression, releasing some of the anger will give you more space in which to operate. It is easier to release it is small doses using its energy to help you get things done. It helps to show compassion for your own anger instead of rejecting it or labeling it as wrong. Your anger has had a purpose. Begin to slowly probe why it is you are feeling angry then allow the inner observer to show you the way to take its energy and transform it into compassion.

It is also necessary to feel your fear. When you open up enough to look at your fear directly, then the gripping, paralyzing power of fear can be acknowledged and put aside. Realize that past conditioning has led you to look at each new challenge in a fearful way and had you withdrawing into yourself. Now that you are on the path to total awareness you can see the fear as just one option then choose to let go of it and focus on the result that you desire. Fear will no longer lead you along by the leash.

In the realm of **gratitude and giving,** you have an opportunity to open yourself up to more abundance. In this life we do not really own or possess anything. We may think we own our homes and our cars, but in reality they are just on loan to us. We will lose all that we have in due time. In expressing gratefulness for what we have today, such attention leads to greater expression of our own gifts. When we recognize that we are fortunate to have a loving spouse and healthy, happy children, we find that we no longer find it necessary to get lost in what we think we need to posses in the material realm to be happy. In sharing the love in family relationships and in caring for each other ,we find that our sense of completeness expands daily.

Some folks may be turned off by the idea of **hugs and touch,** thinking that physical boundaries need to be maintained in order to keep a safe emotional distance. When there is so much unclear energy surrounding your emotional life, the last thing that you want to do is to get swallowed up in someone else's emotional issues. The choice becomes easy to just keep your distance, but that choice does not come without a cost. Down deep you know that you are missing out on something and even though it is your own choice, you just can't figure out what it will take to fill you emotionally and spiritually.

When you withhold physical contact from another, you close yourself off to the closeness and interconnected feeling that is shared by an embrace. Through such physical contact so much more is said than what can be conveyed through the spoken word. Some find it difficult to hug an infant because of the attention it brings to the hugger. Holding the baby, they become the center of attention, and some people just can't tolerate this. In feeling so uncomfortable with their own presence, it is a giant step to reach out to someone. In order to feel comfortable making physical contact, it is necessary to first enjoy your own presence. It is necessary to know your own body and realize that your body is also an energetic instrument that can be used to bring you into sacred space.

If you were brought up in a family where a physical show of affection was taboo, it is understandable that you would be uncomfortable with the idea of physical contact. Here again, the first place to start is in the imagination. In your quiet place, see yourself as first being more comfortable with your own presence, then with time and practice, branch out and see yourself comfortable in the presence of others. Visualize yourself first making energetic contact with those in your inner circle, then appropriate physical contact naturally will follow.

Depending on the degree of your personal discomfort in your own presence, you may experience physical sensations that are initially unpleasant once you decide to begin looking inward and start a meditation practice. Areas of blocked energy that were at first consciously shut down will give you your greatest challenges when you decide that it is safe to start allowing the energy to move again. The problem becomes that, when you decide to look at the fear that has held you back up until now, there is physical pain tied into the locked energy. The awareness of that physical pain feeds back into the fear and can amplify it. In order to get through the fear, you have to make a conscious decision to sit with it for as long as you can, realizing that some days it will be easier to remain within the emotion, while other days you will have to drop what you're doing and walk away.

In **insulating against negativity,** it helps to develop an attitude of "old way/new way". In the past when a distressing thought would arise, it was nothing to allow yourself to follow that thought to the end and let it take you into deeper discontent. That was the old way of doing things. Now that you are working on changing conditions in your life, the new way of approaching negative thoughts is to recognize them for what they are—fear thoughts— acknowledge them, then drop them and replace them with positive affirmation.

The truth of the matter is that when you find yourself drowning in negativity, you have a choice to turn your perception of your situation around one hundred and eighty degrees. When you tell yourself that you doubt you will ever get to your goals, it is just as simple to tell yourself that you are confident that you will reach your goals in time. It takes an element of trust in your ability to receive, and a knowing that you deserve all the good that was meant for you and those that you love. Even if you think changing your attitude will not help, try this technique for the next 30 days and watch how things begin to fall into your lap. No one said it would be easy, as it is never easy staying conscious and aware all of the time, but with practice, you will improve.

Everyone should **journal**. The power of the written word to help us unveil our stance on any and every issue cannot be overemphasized. In *The Artist's Way*,[7] Julia Cameron's guide to greater creativity, we are given as one of the basic tools to fostering creativity what she calls the "morning pages." What has worked for her is to write three pages a day in a stream of consciousness format. She advises to put the pen to paper and let the hand follow the mind. Whatever comes up is to be written down: likes, dislikes, fears, and hopes—everything is to be included. It becomes a way to clear the mind and make room for the creative spark that is within each of us.

The emotions and images that arise during these writing exercises will bring up memories that have been long forgotten. The prize is that once they surface, these repressed and dusty memories can be re-examined from our present day consciousness. The added maturity and life experience helps us reframe our beliefs concerning past events and lets us put them into proper perspective.

To get a bit more focused in our writing and taking it a step beyond journaling, it is wise to follow the advice of Henriette Anne Klauser as given in, *Write It Down, Make It Happen*.[8] She tells us that by writing down the specifics of what we would like to experience in our lives we take our desires out of the realm of imagination and move them into a place where they can manifest. It is similar to an engineer designing a bridge. The plan must first be put to paper, organizing all of the structural details and aesthetic attributes, so that it could eventually unfold into reality. She tells us that by writing our desires down on paper, we make a commitment to lining ourselves up with what we need and want.

The easiest way to begin journaling is to do it just as you get up in the morning. At first it will seem like a huge task, thinking that you want to see so many things happen differently in your life, but as you start writing you will find that there are a finite number of items you will be putting to paper. The trick is to look back periodically to discover what the recurrent themes are for you. Ten minutes a day, or as Julia Cameron recommends, three pages a day is plenty to start. Aside from this, the habit of writing a daily to-do list of things to accomplish is the surest way to get at least 80% of what you need to get done. It only takes a couple of minutes to organize your thoughts on paper, yet this simple activity will save you brain power in the long run as you will not have to keep juggling what needs to be done next on the front burner. For other tips on how to organize your time and your life, which will help reduce stress, see David Allen's *Getting Things Done: The Art of Stress-Free Productivity*.[9]

When it comes to **keep on keeping on,** what is required of us is to practice the virtue of persistence or determination. This is not to say that we do as Nike says when we hear "Just Do It," because our determination has to be coupled with the other virtues of patience, hope, and courage. There will be obstacles that will tempt us to give up and just drop our goals, but by practicing and exercising these virtues, we will make it to the other shore. It will do us well to remember what Donald DeMarco tells us in *The Heart of Virtue: Lessons from Life and Literature Illustrating the Beauty and Value of Moral Character:*

"Determination without patience is impetuosity; without hope, it is blindness. If it is not wedded to discernment, it is mere fanaticism; and if it is not united with courage, it is nothing more than stubbornness. Finally, in the absence of fidelity," (to your purpose), "determination is no more virtuous than compulsive behavior."[10]

So, it is possible to **keep on keeping on** without burning out, as long as we remain balanced in all tasks and take advantage of natural breaks in the action. To go along any other way with open throttle, determination and resolve will only lead to exhaustion and frustration. Learn to feel the natural ebb and flow of all phenomenon.

The 12th happiness habit has to do with our ability to **lighten up and laugh**. Lin Yutang, Chinese philosopher and author recognized, even in the early 1900s, that many of us take life too seriously. He tells us that our seriousness is what leads to troubles. As a remedy for our difficulties, it is beneficial to look on the lighter side of things, as he speaks the following words of advice; "For a sense of humor changes the quality and character of our entire cultural life."[11] Tied up in all of our deep thoughts, it is as if there is no room for *right thought*, as Thich Nhat Hanh describes in *The Heart of the Buddha's Teaching*.[12]

In practicing right thought, we have to realize that thought is the mind's ways of communicating. What we think on all day is where we will go. Allowing yourself to insert laughter into your day, even in the face of adversity, gives you the space required to look at things from a healthier perspective. Though there are conditions that we live by and are influenced by stemming from every past experience we have had, we all have the freedom of choice to direct our thoughts, feelings, and emotions to the higher path.

Notes: Conditions We Live By

1. Csikszentmihalyi, M, *Flow: The Psychology of Optimal Experience* (New York, HarperPerennial 1990), p. 4.

2. His Holiness the Dalai Lama & Cutler, H., *The Art of Happiness at Work* (New York Riverhead Books 2003), pp. 117-138.

3. Finny, M. & Dasch, D, *Find Your Calling, Love Your Life* (Simon & Shuster, 1998). Cited in Brown, T., "A New Breed of Work Force Demands a New Breed of Manager."

From *Managing Yourself for the Career You Want*, (Boston, Harvard Business School Press 2004), pp. 31-39.

4. Mueller, MK, *Taking Care of Me: The Habits of Happiness* (Omaha, Insight Inc 1996), p.69.

5. Tolle, E, *The Power of Now: A Guide to Spiritual Enlightenment* (Novato, California, New World Library 1999), pp. 84-85.

6. Robbins, A. *Awakening the Giant Within* (New York, Simon & Schuster 1991), pp. 200-226.

7. Cameron, J, *The Artists Way: A Spiritual Path to Higher Creativity* (New York, G.P. Putnam's Sons 1992), pp.9-18.

8. Klauser, H. A, *Write It Down, Make It Happen: Knowing What You Want and Getting It!* (New York, Simon & Schuster 2000).

9. Allen, D, *Getting Things Done: The Art of Stress-Free Producitvity*, (New York, Penguin Books 2001).

10. DeMarco, D, *The Heart of Virtue: Lessons from Life and Literature Illustrating the Beauty and Value of Moral Character*, (San Francisco, Ignatius Press 1996), pp.59-61.

11. Cited in "On Humor" by Lin Yutang from *Words to Live By: Selected and Interpreted by Ninety-six Eminent Men and Women*. Edited by William Nichols, (New York, Simon & Schuster, 1949), pp. 53-54.

12. Right Thought is one of the conditions found in the Eight Fold Path one must follow to attain enlightenment. Thich Nhat Hanh, *The Heart of the Buddha's Teaching, Transforming Suffering into Peace, Joy, and Liberation*, (New York, Broadway Books, 1998), pp. 59-63

CHAPTER 5

How to Study Compassion

Affliction is such a harsh word, yet we are all afflicted in one way or another. In deciding to develop compassion toward yourself and others, a new paradigm has to emerge and be developed. No longer will archaic ways of seeing things be adequate to meet your needs. The field of consciousness must and will expand. In recognizing suffering, in whatever realm it may be, and deciding to do something about it, the stage is set for transformation.

Lost in thought and consumed by drama, it is incomprehensible to appreciate the depth of suffering others endure. Imagine a 43-year-old happily married man, around five feet seven inches tall, one hundred and sixty pounds, father of a healthy 4-year-old boy, who works the land as a farmer. He is someone who everyone thinks is wonderful. Seven years ago he had a relatively small skin cancer (melanoma) removed from his back, had treatment, then kept up with yearly chest x-rays and blood work. The nurse calls him back the day after a chest x-ray telling him that the doctor has ordered a CAT scan because there was a new suspicious 1 cm lung nodule. He finds himself going back to the doctor's 360 days early after the doc calls him personally to come in and discuss the findings.

He knows it's not good as he recalls the details the oncologist gave him seven years ago. It keeps going through his mind: "If this cancer had spread, it would be bad because chemotherapy really doesn't work that well in this disease". Now he has to hear all of this again and he can't believe this is happening. He is told that it would be prudent to get a biopsy, so that no bridges are burned in case a new treatment protocol opens up in the very near future. He listens to the dismal role that current therapy plays in his stage of the cancer and his heart sinks to deeper depths as he thinks about his four-year-old son.

This scene is played out all over the world for those suffering from cancer, heart disease, (which also has a propensity to leave its victims debilitated), HIV, and many of the myriad of health conditions to which we are all prone. These examples are not given to suggest that those individuals with a medical illness are the recipients of the greatest suffering. We each understand the meaning of loss. As we get older we lose our youth and for many of us, our health. We lose the idealism we once had and cannot hide the cynicism as we watch misdirected efforts come to naught. When the children grow up we lose our previous relationship with them as exemplified by the empty nest syndrome. Many children lose secure parental relationships to divorce, and have to recalculate and re-sculpt their sense of identity, now shifting and falling into the category of the child of divorced parents. No one is exempt from suffering, and as a protective mechanism, elaborate defense patterns and coping mechanisms are constructed then vigilantly protected by a never resting unconscious. What remains is the repetitive question: "Why am I so tired?"

In a recent interview, Jon Kabat-Kinn, founding director of the Center for Mindfulness in Medicine, Health Care, and Society at the University of Massachusetts Medical School, tells us the next step we must take to become more mindful. With broad brush strokes he states the following: "We need to know more about the science of compassion, the science of empathy, the science of acceptance as well as the art of compassion, the art of empathy, and the art of acceptance."[1] This is an incredibly tall order to fill especially in relation to the amount of time we allow ourselves to feel compassionate during our busy days.

We have to question ourselves and ask what conditions would lead us to a place where we would even consider such a challenge? In today's world a common response might be: what's in it for me? The path of the rest of our lives hinges on our decision to take these steps. Taking a closer look at the charge given to us by Jon Kabot-Zinn, we find that we all have the necessary materials to work with. The natural resources for such growth have been handed down to us through our family DNA and through our nurturing, by way of all of the unique experiences we have had. All of the frustrations we have ever experienced become grist for the mill.

In order to take the first step toward investing energies in the study of compassion it is necessary to examine the internal and external motivating factors. If your life is in a shambles, it is an easy decision to devote more time to self-study and increasing awareness.

On the other hand, if you are mostly satisfied with the way your life is going and can't see yourself functioning in any other capacity, then you probably don't need to do anything different at this time. If this is the case, it is helpful to initiate a quest for compassionate living as the insights revealed may help a loved one, a friend, or an acquaintance. It will also bring contentment and greater satisfaction into your daily living. If the intention is to help move another from suffering, compassion is actively being expressed. This is not to intimate that you should to try to solve everyone's problems, but you may help another come to acceptance and then fruitful action.

If you find yourself losing your patience more often than not, waking up with a sense of dread, feeling more edgy and cranky, or not willing to give up your struggles, then it is time to begin the work of developing greater compassion for yourself. The decision to begin this study may be viewed as selfish, but this is not the case. To take care of yourself is the most courageous and noble responsibility you can undertake. It is the primordial step in developing a genuine, healthy connection with others. It is an act of giving to actually begin working on your issues. In doing so you change things so that others do not have to deal with your foibles and you begin clearing the way for genuine communication which is conducive to growth and health. Clear communication conveys your need at this moment. When you know what you need and are able to ask for it, such knowledge and wisdom displaces previously learned dysfunction.

When we begin to undertake the study of any subject, it is first necessary to define what the objective of study will be. Are we going to spend time learning new subject matter just to sound educated and show off, or will we go into this activity with the higher goal of coming away with greater wisdom, and exercising that which we have learned? In the study of compassion, one of the byproducts is a general softening of the attitude. This spills over into how we relate to those around us. A sense of ease moves in like fluffy, soft, billowing clouds on a spring afternoon. Much of the previous intensity, impatience, and dark background energy of anger transforms into acceptance and understanding. Your concept of time will alter and as a result there will be more room in your day to do the things that fulfill you.

Setting the groundwork for what you would like to see happen is not only practical, but also smart. As you set the goal of acting with greater compassion, the intention leads to a metamorphosis resulting in the expression of a living virtue that will positively affect the lives of others. Instead of peering into some unknown distant future, you will, with increasing frequency, ask yourself ,what is the best and most effective thing to be done right now? With this information you will know the next step to take and eventually the question will broaden to ask, what is the best and most effective step to take now that will benefit all parties involved.

As you learn to listen more deeply to your inner guidance, you discover it helpful to write things down. It is best to do this within a few minutes of your insight as we all recognize that thoughts are fleeting, and who knows how long it will be before these ideas will arise again. As you set aside more time for yourself, solitude will show you where your dominant thoughts reside. Use the time to make friends with yourself and deal with issues of procrastination and the path will open in front of you. When you find yourself stuck in a particular place, ask yourself why these images keep coming back to slow you down. You will find the original thought was sealed in your belief system many years ago, at a time when you did not have a full grasp of the meaning of your situation or circumstance. You did your best at the time, but now it is necessary to restructure your thoughts. Bringing the mind-body connection into a symbiotic relationship eventually leads to an overall greater sense of ease.

In order to see new points of focus we need a way to gauge the changes that are occurring. What we are looking for are changes in perceptions, of seeing the bigger picture in our lives, and recognizing a palpable decrease in our desire to keep holding on. There are things we can do to track our attachments. It will take some effort, but if we view this exercise in the same vein as the morning pages that Julia Cameron describes in *The Artists Way*, the activity will soon become a useful method for keeping us in the realm of skillful thought and action.

The following are a set of sample questions you can ask yourself when it comes to monitoring changes in your feelings and thinking. As a way to quantify your answers, and view them in a more precise manner, it is helpful to score your answers between zero and ten, with zero being never having the experience and ten being that you always see things happening in the described manner.

How to Measure Compassion

How high is your anxiety level today?
0   1   2   3   4   5   6   7   8   9   10

How is your sense of ease today?
0   1   2   3   4   5   6   7   8   9   10

What degree of patience with others are you experiencing?
0   1   2   3   4   5   6   7   8   9   10

How would you grade your present awareness, or the amount of time you spent living in the now today?
0   1   2   3   4   5   6   7   8   9   10

How much time did you spend looking to place blame?
0   1   2   3   4   5   6   7   8   9   10

Did you allow others to feel "OK" today?
0   1   2   3   4   5   6   7   8   9   10

How many acts of kindness did you do today?
0   1   2   3   4   5   6   7   8   9   10

How well connected do you feel today?
0   1   2   3   4   5   6   7   8   9   10

Did you have any demonstrations of friendliness?
0   1   2   3   4   5   6   7   8   9   10

Degree of grasping:
To old ideas
0   1   2   3   4   5   6   7   8   9   10

To material objects
0   1   2   3   4   5   6   7   8   9   10

To relationships
0   1   2   3   4   5   6   7   8   9   10

Much of the unease that we feel on a daily basis originates from our feelings of anxiety. With all of the demands placed on us from all directions, it is difficult to feel comfortable in our own skin. Eckhart Tolle, in *The Power of Now* describes, something called the "pain body." He tells us that we all have one. It is the physical and emotional pain we experience that has been handed down through generations. He tells us that the pain we create is always some form of non-acceptance. It is our way to resist what is.[2] Knowing that the "pain body" exists is the first step in understanding our challenge in coping with it effectively. It is an energy that can come upon us at any time and make us feel uncomfortable. The concept stems from the idea that the sins of the father are the sins of the son, yet does not imply that we actually pay for the sins of our fathers. Instead we suffer because of their sins (in this instance their lack of living in the now and practicing Right Thought, Right Action, Right Concentration, Right Livelihood, and the remainder of the Eight Fold Path).

As we grow, we watch every move our parents make, initially learning everything from them. We see the world just as they do, but do not possess the same depth of understanding that they have. As the Dutch proverb states, "De appel valt niet ver van de boom" ("The apple does not fall far from the tree.")[3] It is not until the teenage years that we really begin to see things differently and begin to come to our own conclusions. This is actually part of our ongoing problem because the conclusions we come to are many times final and seem to be set in stone. Unless we were taught early on that no conclusion is the truth, we will go on to live out the "pain body" we have been handed down. The common practice of blaming our parents for the difficulties we face is rooted in our lack of recognition or understanding of the "pain body."

Needless to say, no one really likes their "pain body." It is only natural to shy away from something that causes so much discomfort and pain, but in order to understand it and grow with it, we have to be willing to courageously open up that box. The same thing holds for looking at the pain that others experience. Much pain and anxiety is rooted in an individual's sense of shame. In order to be compassionate, we have to be able and willing to understand another's source of shame, but we are not capable of doing even that until we acknowledge our own "pain body."

Webster's Third New International Dictionary describes shame as, "a painful emotion caused by consciousness of guilt, shortcoming, or impropriety in one's own behavior." It can also be explained as "dishonor, disgrace, or something worthy of strong censure."[4] A life lived shrouded in shame cuts off the capacity to feel. In disconnecting and losing touch with basic needs as belonging, recognition, and acceptance, daily function becomes one of survival mode. When experiencing pain, every action becomes one of removing oneself from the source of the pain. This may take the form of any one of the addictive behaviors such as workaholism, alcoholism, and in families can lead to a multitude of dysfunctional behaviors as described by John Bradshaw in *Healing the Shame that Binds You*.[5] He tells us that control is the major defense strategy for shame. Growing up in this environment, families may find the predominant emotion expressed is one form of anger. After a day at work, coming home and finding the house a mess may lead to outbursts of anger. The environment is out of control, and there is just too much activity, energy, and noise coming from the children. The peace contemplated all day long is nonexistent, and this leads to an even deeper sense of frustration. Feeling powerless and defeated, the children become the object of our overwhelming emotions. All that was wanted and deserved was a little peace and quiet, but because of an inability to ask for what is needed, everyone suffers.

A common manifestation of internalized shame is perfectionism. As Bradshaw explains there is a need to "always be right in everything you do ... The fear and avoidance of the negative is the organizing principle of life...No one ever measures up."[6] To live under such pressure day-to-day and year-to-year leads to further harm and self-destruction. With this heavy burden, the heart hardens leaving no room for the softness of compassion. How can an individual be compassionate to themselves when all of their energy goes into maintaining defenses against overwhelming feelings of inadequacy?

Further efforts to hide shame leave one with no alternative but to blame others for their misfortunes and short-comings. Unable to effectively deal with failure, the threat to their belief of perfection is intolerable. It becomes easy to divert attention away from the self and find a multitude of reasons why others can take the blame for a perceived failure. In this way personal responsibility is denied and others are viewed as objects of scorn. No wonder there is pervasive difficulty communicating needs to others in an honest manner.

Bradshaw continues to tell us that shame keeps us from expressing our human potential by demanding that we no longer perceive, think, feel, desire, or imagine the way that would lead to creative action. This is because our image of perfection keeps us bound by its parameters. When we are hurt it is natural and healthy to express anger and disappointment, but when we live with the image of perfection, it is that image itself that keeps us from expressing our feelings. We still feel the anger and may even lash out at loved ones. The emotions are there but the appropriate expression is inhibited, thus we are left at a loss for what we are feeling and are labeled as being cranky, or worse, immature.

In reading *Healing the Shame that Binds You*, it is only reasonable to do so in small doses. As the conditions described within hit home, there may be an overpowering sense of futility as many maladaptive thoughts and behaviors are brought into full view. Until now, feelings were hidden from yourself and others. If one was never taught that we are all worthy of expressing our feelings, or if one was programmed to believe that needs and desires are not to be shared, the mold is set for dysfunction. If the predominant emotion expressed in a household is raw anger one unfortunately will have little idea of how to deal with it effectively and in a way that it can be of productive service. Fortunately, compassion transforms anger and fear into acceptance and peace.

Kat Duff, in *The Alchemy of Illness,* tells us of her struggle with chronic fatigue and immune dysfunction syndrome. In her writings she takes us back to the days of the 16th century alchemists explaining that their philosophy was "that physical decay is the beginning of the "Great Work": spiritual transformation." She describes the four qualities that alchemists tell us must be present to help us find the basic matter than we can work with for spiritual transformation: "(1) It is ordinary and found everywhere; (2) people are often revolted by it; (3) it has many names and faces but only one essence; (4) it is boundless, consuming, and overwhelming."[7]

In our efforts to get through the day, much of the time we actively exert energy in our attempt to avoid our own problems. Since we view our own problems as something to avoid and turn a blind eye to, why in the world would we want to even consider looking at the problems that others face? One major reason to open up to the suffering of others is that this is exactly the direction we need to move in order to heal. The dance to health will take us from the fumbling of an infant, to the clumsiness of an adolescent, and eventually to the waltz past middle age and beyond. Certainly there will be issues that we will not want to look at, but why continue on in a life that finds us half asleep to reality, and numb from the pain, when we can open our eyes and begin to see the connecting threads that we all share?

Since many of us spend so much time on the job, our work offers the perfect place to express compassion. In *Toxic Emotions at Work*, Peter J. Frost brings to our attention the fact that not everyone we deal with is motivated by the same compassionate standards. He reminds us that, "malice, interpersonal incompetence, and insensitivity are all potential characteristics of people- whether or not they hold management or leadership positions."[8] He describes what he refers to refers to as "toxin handlers," or those individuals within an organization who voluntarily deal with the pain that results as a matter of carrying on the business of the day. Their roles are to offer compassionate help and practical input to stressed employees.[9] Many times, the one's who are being compassionate are not even aware of the service they are providing. Of greater concern is the idea that the organizational leadership has no idea of what is going on either.

In today's climate, with the bottom line on the top of everyone's consciousness (especially those in leadership roles), there is a high degree of insensitivity to the plight of workers undergoing emotional turmoil. In their intense drive to achieve business success or personal recognition, many company leaders are blind to the emotional needs of their peers and staff. This can be as extreme as a partner in a medical practice abusing drugs to cope with his work load, resulting in his death. Along the way to this disaster, there are subtle hints that something is not right. The partner runs his car into a tree on his way home from the hospital after a night call, or he slurs his speech one morning while speaking to the charge nurse on rounds. Such behavior is written off as having a bad night on call. Only after the irreparable damage has been done are the real questions allowed out in the open for discussion. As Frost tells us,

"Some managers cannot separate work from the emotional needs of their staff. They have trouble identifying with a staff member's distress, or else they operate from a belief that everyone's emotions (including their own) should be checked at the office door. Such managers don't understand why anyone's personal life, even emotional pain, should take priority over workplace tasks and commitments. As a result, they respond insensitively to a colleague's cry for help—and lose the loyalty and willingness of that person to go the extra mile for the manager or the organization."[10]

The message to the one who is suffering is clear and is akin to the notion: "if you can't stand the heat, then get out of the kitchen." Instead of admonishing individuals in such a situation, the organization has the opportunity to broaden its scope of services. By having greater sensitivity to the needs of not only its clients, but also the work staff, the bottom line will improve. In addition, in taking the time and energy to investigate the emotional needs of the staff, greater loyalty is shown. With an increased sense of connectedness, there are more opportunities for states of flow, and thus greater efficiency and productivity. Instead of perceiving a troubled fellow human as a problem, the corrective measure is to allow such individuals to work where their greatest service lies.

The degree of sensitivity expressed by those in the throes of difficulty can be used to bring out the real issues of your consumers as well as employees. In a sense, such immeasurable though palpable emotion allows allows for deeper connections between individuals. Making it safe for employees to move in this direction will decrease the stress all around. An added benefit is a growing reputation of caring on the part of your organization.

At this point you may question why anyone would ever want to play the role of a toxin handler. As Frost points out, there are many reasons - some more harmful to the handler than others. The individual who has a low self-esteem and high emotional sensitivity will perform above and beyond for the simple reason of gaining approval. This is the most dangerous situation in which to be, as the handler has given up his own power as he looks to others for validation. Everything is done for external reasons, and there is usually a great deal of second-guessing concerning what could have been done better. Because of intense sensitivity, toxin handlers have trouble letting go of the problems of the day. Even when sleep comes, dreams involve work situations. Up at 3 in the morning, tossing and turning, worrying about the challenges of the day ahead, it is no wonder the morning is greeted with an all too familiar feeling of exhaustion.

Basically, the best way to deal with and start to move away from the role of a toxin handler is to begin to develop compassion for yourself. It is necessary to understand that to take care of others, one must first take care of the self. This means examining your situation and looking at the circumstances where you find yourself getting hooked into another's pain. It means keeping your finger on your own pulse and realizing that you need to schedule breaks so you can recharge your batteries. Exercising limits by saying "no" to certain requests will do much to relieve stress, and just because you tell someone "no," that doesn't mean that you can't or won't help them later.

In developing compassion for yourself, it is necessary to know how to ask for what you need. If you find yourself on the road to burnout and you don't know how to ask for a break, you will get a break, but it may not be the kind that you really want. The practices of yoga and meditation will help you focus on what you really need and will help you bring your life into greater balance. This is not to say that all of your days will be perfectly balanced, but on the sine curve of life, you will be working closer to center if you choose the middle road.

Building on the work of others, Frost tells us that toxin handlers need to work on four different areas of their lives. They need to 1) strengthen their physical capacity, 2) boost their emotional capacity, 3) regenerate their mental capacity, and 4) build their spiritual capacity.[11] To strengthen physical capacity sounds easy, but many of us do not carve out the time to do so on a consistent basis. For me, yoga is the mainstay of my exercise program, though for the past five years I have focused more on the restorative poses than the challenging ones, like handstand or headstand. I know I should get to the YMCA pool more often, but family time is a priority. Others like to jog, take brisk walks, kayak, and bicycle, play tennis or racquetball, or just work out. Physical strength will translate into greater self-confidence, so choose whatever activity you like and muster up the discipline to stick with it.

To strengthen your emotional capacity, it helps to stay keenly aware of where you invest your emotional energy, for failing to do so will leave you drained. Begin the study of how you react to the events of your day on a gut-level. Start to pay attention to how the words of others and their intonations affect you. If you discover that being in close proximity to someone leaves you drained, it is time to consider spending less time with them or taking steps to learn techniques that will prevent the energy drain. One technique is to simply remain grounded in the presence of that individual. This can be achieved by imagining a thick cord running from your feet to the center of the earth. Keep this image in mind instead of placing all of your focus and concentration on the source of your energy drain.

Mira Kirshenbaum, in *The Emotional Energy Factor,* gives us plenty of tips on how to boost our emotional energy. She advises that we stop buying into other's expectations for us.[12] When we are able to put the fear down and look at our lives with compassion, a picture of impermanence flashes across the screen of the mind and gives us a hint that maybe we should start doing what we have always wanted to do.

The next suggestion Kirshenbaum gives to strengthen your emotional capacity is to give your life meaning. For many of us, the grueling road has taken the shine out of life. Like robots, we stiffly rise from bed in the morning and shuffle. The spark is gone and we haven't taken the time to ask why. Show compassion for yourself by asking again.

The question for many of us becomes: What exactly do we have to ask for to begin a renewed search for meaning?

James Allen eloquently gives us a hint of what must be done to find meaning. He tells us the following:

"Only by much searching and mining are gold and diamonds obtained, and man can find every truth connected with his being if he will dig deep into the mine of his soul; and that he is the maker of his character, the molder of his life, and the builder of his destiny, he may unerringly prove, if he will watch, control, and alter his thoughts, tracing their effects upon himself, upon others, and upon his life and circumstances, linking cause and effect by patient practice and investigation, and utilizing his every experience, even to the most trivial, everyday occurrence, as a means of obtaining that knowledge of himself which is Understanding, Wisdom, Power. In this direction, as in no other, is the law absolute that "He that seeketh findeth; and to him that knocketh it shall be opened"; for only by patience, practice, and ceaseless importunity can a man enter the Door of the Temple of Knowledge.[13]

Neal Stephenson, a science fiction writer, talks about the *Star Wars* craze and how "geeks" know all of the ins and outs of who the good guys are and who the bad guys are. Many of us who watch *Stars Wars* are entertained and enjoy the zoned out feeling of getting lost in the action and suspense. The movie takes us away from our daily troubles. Geeks see the movies and study the books to learn more about the culture about which George Lucas has been writing for the past twenty-five years. We all know what geeks are, but many of us do not know what they do. According to Stephenson, they are individuals who study the details of a subject.[14] Ask a Star Wars geek anything about the *Star Wars* movies or books and they will tell you *ad infinitum* more than you want to know and maybe more than you would understand.

Unless you have also read the *Star Wars* books, you would never know that Princess Leia and Hans Solo had a child they named Anakin Solo, or that the stormtrooper whose armor Luke appropriates is numbered TK-421. A greater challenge is to list all of the Rebel pilots who die over the Death Star by name and squadron number. For the Star Wars fans they are as follows: Red Leader, Red Three (Biggs Darklighter), Red Four (John D.), Red Six (Porkins), Red Ten, Red Eleven, Gold Leader (Dutch), Gold Two (Tiree), Gold Five (Pops).[15] Query a non-Star Wars geek about the movies and they will tell you many times that they are not sure where what fits in or who the good guys and who the bad guys are. The question becomes: How do we get "geekish" about the study of compassion?

The article, *Compassion in Organizational Life*, written by Jason M. Kanov et al., gives us a deeper look at some of the operational definitions of compassion.[16] Their elaboration on the subject helps us form a clearer picture of this otherwise nebulous virtue. They, and others before them, support the opinion that compassion has to be viewed in the context of interactions with others. They see this virtue as a dynamic process and go further to explain it as a set of sub-processes that include noticing, feeling, and responding to another's pain. The first hurdle to overcome in acting in a compassionate way is to come to the realization that the pain associated with change is a legitimate pain.[17]

Just because we cannot see or measure another's pain, does not mean it is not real. Even in the medical clinic, many patients who experience pain have anxiety over relating their pain and "convincing" the doctor that they actually have pain. Useful clinical indicators used to support the presence of significant pain are the vital signs.

If the heart rate is over 100, the blood pressure is higher than usual, or if the individual appears to be in distress: wearing a facial grimace, having beads of sweat about the forehead, or experiencing difficulty with concentration, then it is easy to justify giving the patient pain medicine.

On the other hand, if the individual converses with ease, has normal vital signs, and is without obvious distress, the decision to dispense narcotic pain medicines may be withheld. The reality is that many people have chronic pain from arthritis, past injuries, contractures, myofascial pain syndromes, post-surgical causes, or post radiation problems. They have learned how to function day to day, tolerating their pain to various degrees, and rely on the pain medicines on their "bad" days.

Under the pressure to perform at work and to meet quotas, our minds are so tied up in getting the job done that in many instances, there is insufficient attention allotted to recognizing the plight of others. This is especially so on an emotional level. If, because of harried conditions, we are forced into a position of decreased sensitivity and receptivity, everyone suffers. If we are working at 110% most of the time, or dealing with chronic fatigue because of high work loads and expectations, then there is simply not enough energy to even consider the emotional burdens of others. There are levels of compassion that can be touched upon based on individual capacities.

People are born with different temperaments, some so sensitive that they need to avoid the pain of others at all costs. These are individuals who come home from work drained, go to bed drained, do not sleep well, and wake up drained. They find their energy in solitude. Aware of this, they need to take care of their needs, find work that allows them to express their inner drives and desires, spend limited time with others, and acknowledge to themselves that this is how they function at their best.

Others are "people people", sometimes to the degree that they cannot tolerate any time alone. They blossom in groups, they energize by spending time with others, and sometimes they talk so much that they are exhausting to listen to. They need to do what is best for them, but to add balance to their lives, it is useful to carve out small snippets of time to think on their own.

When we take the time to notice the pain of another, this simple act allows the sufferer some relief. Many times the burden leaves its mark as feelings of inadequacy, isolation, and disorientation. To look beyond what another can do for you and open your heart to the pain of another, you broaden your world. The next time you notice someone in distress, slow down and ask yourself what it was at first that cued you in to their plight. Was it that you had a similar kind of pain in the past and their movement, speech, or actions mirrored what you felt during that period? Do you tend to notice distress in those whom you like and only those in your inner circle, or do you leave yourself open to feeling the turmoil of all who are in proximity? If the latter is the case, you may need to work on tightening your emotional boundaries, but only to a degree, since it is humane to feel. There are healthy ways to deal with the pain of others, and one of the best ways to work on this is through a daily meditation and yoga practice.

In feeling for another, we have to watch that we do not take on an attitude that the world is always unfair. It is important to steer away from a sense of bitterness about the reality of suffering. Here, it will do us well to remember that we all suffer, but when looking at the overall picture, it is how we view our suffering that will dictate whether it brings us down or brings us closer to others.

In order to respond to the suffering of another, we have to have an inner confidence that we can get through what is put before us. Fortitude is not unthinkingly going into a situation and bullying yourself through it, but instead it is an inner knowing that no matter what happens you will make it to the other shore. There will be resolution for all problems in their own time. A word of recognition, a short note of acknowledgement, or a word of encouragement may be more helpful to one who suffers than you know. It may be just the thing that allows the pain to subside long enough for the sufferer to have a reasonable day. It takes a willingness to step out of your own world and move into unstable space to open to those in need. Begin to look for ways to expand your consciousness in this direction, and your sense of connectedness will grow.

The question arises concerning how we get an organization to recognize one's pain when we have had to deny the pain just to keep working. This is where the work of increasing self-awareness and learning about the mind-body connection through yoga, meditation, guided imagery, acupuncture, counseling, and spiritual practice come into play. Until we, as individuals, allow ourselves to take a look at what is really going on, we will suffer in the darkness. Only when we are able to put people before objects, performance, and materials will we live in greater health.

With all of the emotional and behavioral undercurrents of our consciousness, it is not unreasonable to think that we may never get to the bottom of our suffering. The majority of today's health care institutions still view individuals from the perspective of finding and fixing a disease. There is a place for this kind of medicine, as it has helped millions pull away from the grip of suffering. It is fortunate that our federal government is now aggressively funding the National Center for Complimentary and Alternative Medicine. In fiscal year 1992, Congress funded the then Office of Alternative Medicine with 2 million. By 1998 that number was increased to $19.5 million. In 1999, the Office of Alternative Medicine became the National Center for Complementary and Alternative Medicine (NCCAM) and was funded with $50 million. In fiscal year 2005, Congress appropriated $123.1 million to the NCCAM for use in research, training, and teaching fellowships.[18]

In a review comparing how Complimentary and Alternative Medicine (CAM) consultations differ from Conventional Medicine (CM) consultations, Adrian Furnham, Ph.D. explains that CAM consultations give more time to patients, there is more touch involved, the history taking is holistic/affective versus specific/behavioral for CM. During CAM consultations, the language used is described as healing, holistic, and subjective. It is geared toward obtaining a personal history and focused around the idea of wellness. This is in contrast to the language used in CM, which is focused on curing. It is objective, based on case histories, and is centered on illness.

With CAM the patient's role is that of a consumer, while with CM, their role is that of a sick person. Decision making is shared in CAM, whereas in CM the doctor plays a paternalistic role. The bedside manner of a CAM practitioner is charismatic and empathetic, versus cool and professional for the CM practitioner.[19] If we can integrate some of the CAM principles into conventional medicine over time, we will find an expanding role of compassion in the practice of caring for others.

CAM is currently defined as a group of diverse medical and health care systems, practices, and products that are not presently considered to be part of conventional medicine. Complimentary medicine is used along with conventional medicine while alternative medicine is used in place of conventional medicine. Reports on the number of users of CAM vary, but a report published in the November 11, 1998, issue of the *Journal of the American Medical Association* found that CAM use among the general public increased from 33.8 percent in 1990 to 42.1 percent in 1997.[20] In 1990 and 1997 at Harvard Medical School, Eisenberg demonstrated the breadth of American interest in CAM. He found a 47% increase in total visits to CAM providers during this time period. The number of visits increased from 427 million in 1990 to 629 million in 1997. In both survey years, the number of visits to CAM providers surpassed the total visits to all U.S. primary care physicians. The amount spent on these therapies was $14 billion in 1990 and $27 billion in 1997.[21]

Americans are crying out for help. Mainstream medicine is good for what it does, but there is still a great deal of suffering that is not being addressed. As more research is done through NCCAM clinical trials, hopefully the practitioners of complementary and alternative medicine will work side by side with the doctors of conventional medicine and we will reap the benefits of both worlds. As we do, the expression of compassion will be a given, and as we find a place for this virtue in our daily lives we cannot help but learn more about it.

Notes: How to Study Compassion

1. Interview with Jon Kabat-Zinn, Ph.D. by Karolyn A. Gazella, "Bringing Mindfulness To Medicine." *Alternative Therapies in Health and Medicine,* May/June 2005, Vol. 11, No.3, pp.57-64.

2. Tolle, E, *The Power of Now,* (New World Library, Novato CA, 1999), pp. 27-38.

3. Taken from Wikiquote. http://en.wikiquote.org/wiki/Dutch_proverbs#T.

4. From *Webster's Third New International Dictionary of the English Language Unabridged,* (Merriam-Webster, Springfield, Massachusetts, 1993).

5. Bradshaw, J, *Healing the Shame that Binds You.* (Health Communications, Deerfield Beach, Florida, 1988), pp. 39-41.

6. Ibid. p. 40.

7. Duff, Kat, *The Alchemy of Illness.* (Bell Tower, New York, 1993), pp.79-80.

8. Frost, P, *Toxic Emotions at Work.* (Harvard Business School Press, Boston, 2003), p.50.

9. Ibid. p.16.

10. Ibid. p. 42.

11. Loehr, J, & Schwartz, T, *The Making of a Corporate Athlete,* (Harvard Business Review, January 2001), pp. 122, 120-128, 123, as described by Frost, P, *Toxic Emotions at Work.* (Harvard Business School Press, Boston, 2003), pp. 107-132.

12. Kirshenbaum, M, *The Emotional Energy Factor: The Secrets High-Energy People Use to Beat Emotional Fatigue,* (Delacorte Press, New York, 2003), pp. 19-36.

13. Allen, J, As A Man Thinketh, (Grosset & Dunlap, New York), pp. 7-8.

14. Neal Stephenson is a science fiction writer who has authored the 1999 bestselling *Cryptonomicon,* about present-day high-tech entrepreneurs mixed with World War II adventures, and cryptography. The material presented was quoted from the *New York Times* OP-ED section published 6/17/05.

15. For more *Stars Wars* trivia see, *Jedimaster Simon H. Lee's Trivia Challenge* at http://www.theforce.net/jedicouncil/trivia/swtrivia.asp.

16. Kanov, J, Maitlis, S, Worline, M, Dutton, J, Frost, P, & Lilius, J. *Compassion In Organizational Life.* The complete article can be found on the web at http://www.compassionlab.org.

17. Dutton, J. "Breathing Life into Organizational Studies," *Journal of Management Inquiry,* 12. 1-19, 2003, as cited in *Compassion in Organizational Life.* See note #16, p.4.

18. The yearly appropriations of funds to the Office of Alternative Medicine and the National Center for Complementary and Alternative Medicine can be

found at http://nccam.nih.gov/about/appropriations/index.htm

19. Report from a conference on January 23-24, 2001 in London, England, titled "Can Alternative Medicine Be Integrated into Mainstream Care?" Issues covered can be found at http://nccam.nih.gov/news/pastmeetings/012301/index.htm#2.

20. Information on complimentary medicine and cancer treatment can be found at http://cis.nci.nih.gov/fact/9_14.htm.

21. Eisenberg DM, Davis RB, Ettner L et al."Trends in alternative medicine use in the United States, 1990-1997: Results of a follow-up national survey. *JAMA* 1998; 280: 1569-1575.

CHAPTER 6

Changing Views

Have you ever wondered what is it about this generation of Americans that makes us believe, on one hand, that we want things to change as quickly as possible, and on the other hand, when change does occur, we have difficulty adjusting to it, and resist it with everything we have? Such thinking divides the mind, resulting in misdirected energies working in opposite directions. It makes for a very tired society that lacks clarity and direction.

We all know deep down that change is inevitable and that most change is for the better, but on the surface, where we usually look for answers (more than we would like to admit), there is a general dislike toward change because it forces us to think differently. Change forces us out of our comfort zones. Adapting to change takes effort and plenty of patience, thus when we are looking for and wanting change in our lives, it is difficult to bring about the actual changes that we want. Invested in the drudgery of the day, we get trapped by complaining, we diffuse out energies and then are at a loss when it comes to taking positive steps to bring about the changes we desire.

The question becomes: How do we look for change that does more than usher in fleeting happiness? We need to learn to seek the kind of change that brings meaning into our lives. Wanting change for the sake of change, or because we are bored, is not conducive to lasting fulfillment. External change alone does not result in eternal peace or satisfaction, whereas inner transformation brings us toward lasting peace, contentment, and joy. Just as there are ways of dealing with change that leave us frustrated, there are perspectives to embrace, such as acceptance of impending change, that help us grow in understanding during times of change.

How do you deal with change in your life? If you are dissatisfied, tired of the way things are going, and are ready to seek greater clarity, meaning, and fulfillment, then it is time to consider this question. To be tossed, thrown, and beaten by the tide of change, like an old tire in the ocean, leads to feelings of helplessness, despair, and powerlessness. Resisting the waves of your emotions leaves you and others wondering what will happen next. When your inner compass has been neutralized by listless confusion, spinning, blurred thoughts, and emotional turmoil surrounding change, any sense of control feels far beyond reach. Lacking mastery when it comes to dealing with everyday change, the prospect of impending change is overwhelming. Is this what you want?

When someone is described as being "solid as a rock," we imagine a strong, Herculean individual. We think this is a wonderful and useful trait to have, believing that those blessed have the ability to cope with greater stress than the average person. But to place this label - solid as a rock

- on anyone, paints a picture of rigidity and inflexibility. Trees in nature that have a low center of gravity, a deep root system, and a strong sturdy trunk - like oak trees - are more likely to survive the stress and ravage beatings of a hurricane. On the other hand, trees that are considered the weakest link of the landscape - pine trees - are the ones with a high center of gravity, a dense canopy, a weak trunk, and shallow roots. In the same vein, if we go about our days with dense energy and extremely tough skin, we will be insensitive to our own feelings and the feeling of others. This makes us impervious to the early signs of change so that our awareness is such that only when the signs become obvious, do we notice the change. With this lack of insight, we wonder how things could have turned out the way they did. Tall, slender trees, like pines, are the ones that snap, fall to the ground, and leave only a remnant of their existence that will later be food for bugs and insects.[1] We have the choice to remain flexible and light with our energies, and still remain rooted in the midst of change. This permits us to sense impending change and make the appropriate adjustments along the way. With our conscious intervention, there is a greater probability that the results will be to our liking.

To remain relaxed and open no matter what is going on around us is to be in a position of power. Such a stance gives us the advantage of better knowing what to do next. If we experience turmoil and tense up at the first sign of trouble, our first goal becomes one of seeing the connection, or the hook, that makes us react in the old way. A conscious decision has to be made not to resort back to ineffective, worn-out coping mechanisms. To remain rock-solid prevents the softness that makes the ground fertile for compassion and caring. Over time, the edges of the rock become jagged as trials and tribulations chip away at us, removing what is left of any gentleness we may have known.

In order to ride the wave of change and feel less pain, it is necessary to keep the big picture in mind. As Diane Ackerman tells us in *An Alchemy of Mind*, we rely on both sides of our brain to help us make decisions. If the choice was solely that of the left side of the brain, with its continual and incessant internal conversations, we would end up in a dialogue that would leave us more confused than we already are. No one likes to be in the same room as an incessant talker, lost in their own thought, showing no concern for the listener. As Ackerman explains, it takes an integrated, balanced brain to come to a conclusion concerning our choices, and even though we have to deal with the left brain's ceaseless rambling, individuals who are left brain dominant have a better self-image and higher levels of enthusiasm for life. Right brain dominant individuals tend to experience more bouts of depression and have a harder time getting over depression than left brain dominants.[2] So it would appear that being left brain dominant would put one at an advantage when it comes to making decisions, especially important, life changing decisions.

Knowing where you fit in this schema, it helps to trace back your steps and decipher where your current reactions to change have originated. In doing this, the most difficult part is staying with the discomfort associated with old patterns of thinking and remaining present until you find an effective way to view the changes that will inevitably come. It has been demonstrated that Tibetan Lamas who meditate have greater electrical activity in the left prefrontal cortex of their brains. This portion of the brain has been associated with the positive temperaments that we all crave, such as compassion, ease, confidence, and peace.

The same group of scientists who discovered this took volunteers from a high-tech company and trained them in meditation techniques over an eight week period. At the end of the training, the meditators had greater electrical activity in the left prefrontal cortex than the control group. This group also showed an augmented immune response to the flu vaccine compared to the untrained group.[3]

Studies such as the above show us that we can change our habitual responses to previously perceived uncomfortable or even dangerous situations. We can also make ourselves healthier in the process. It would appear that one would not have to believe that such training actually works, but it takes effort to start the activity and keep it going.

As noted in the psychological literature, there is a relationship between stress and distress. The term "rumination" is used to describe the tendency for individuals to persist in a goal directed activity, or invest their energies toward that goal, until they have either reached their goal or given up on the idea of attaining it.[4] It is one thing to remain focused, but another to act obsessively to the point of going around with tunnel vision. Staying in a persistent mode of intense concentration, we forfeit all that occurs on the periphery of our activity. There is a similar phenomenon that occurs with stargazing. If you try to directly view the star in question, say Betelgeuse in the Orion constellation, even though it is a bright star with a magnitude of 0.45 (though not as bright as Sirius, the brightest star in the sky, with a magnitude of -1.46), it will appear less intense than if you looked at it with your peripheral vision. Forcing yourself to function with too deep a focus, you no longer feel the cool breeze as it passes over tense skin; the baby blue sky above could just as easily be a dark dungeon, and the concerns of others, of which we are an integral part, are the last things on our minds. We can choose to stay so busy, getting into a routine of going to work early and staying late, that we may actually miss one of the seasons.

In choosing to ruminate, we lock ourselves into a thought pattern and cut ourselves off from refreshing change. It is as if we believe without a doubt that we know what is going to happen next in our lives, and in our "knowing," or know-it-all attitude, we close the door to any healthy change and keep going on with business as usual. For events to unfold naturally, there needs to be an element of trust and the old, ever-watchful, vigilant attitude, and any controlling tendencies have to be abandoned. When a seed is planted in the ground, it does not tell the clouds to water it with their nourishing elixir. The clouds will always release their prize when the moisture content exceeds a certain level. The seed does not know that the water will leech away a germinator inhibitor called abscisic acid. The seed has no idea that this hormone is responsible for it's adaptation to stress and that abscisic acid in the cells at the tip of the stem cause the plant to go into a dormant state in cold weather, thus allowing it to survive during the harsh winter months.[5]

We also have hormones that influence the way we behave and feel. They can overpower us and cause us to behave in unexpected and uncharacteristic ways, as demonstrated by the effects of hormones on us during puberty. We have all known a previously responsible teenager who, under the influence of higher levels of testosterone, will stay out all night, unconcerned over what his parents think. This kind of behavior is stressful for both the individual having the experience and the parents. However, it is not only the teenager who suffers the wrath of increased hormone levels. Throughout our lives, hormones continue to affect our moods, responses, and overall health in some very profound ways.

Cortisol is our major stress hormone. It is a steroid hormone with a similar structure to the female and male sex hormones. It is produced by highly organized clumps of tissue that sit on top of each kidney called the adrenals glands. Its regulating stimulator is ACTH (adrenocorticotropin hormone) that is produced by the pituitary gland. The place of residence of this powerful, specialized neuronal tissue is deep within the brain. It sits at the base of the skull in its own protective cavern (the sella turcica). This structure is actually a bony box that was named after the "Turkish saddle", because both have supports in the front and the back. Such an arrangement offers greater protection for this very important gland - a structure that not only mediates ACTH output, but also controls the levels of growth hormone, thyroid hormone, sex hormones, as well as prolactin, a hormone that stimulates the breast to produce milk.[6]

The levels of these hormones are in a state of constant flux, and it has been found that most heart attacks occur in the early morning hours when the levels of cortisol, estrogen, progesterone, and testosterone are at their peak levels.[7] Cortisol levels jump up and kick into effect when our nervous systems sense danger. For the many folks who have difficulty with change, or any other major challenge of the post-traumatic stress disorder type, even when the actual danger is gone, those affected feel and react emotionally and mentally as if the noxious stimuli persist. As a result they live in a hyper-alert state. In such a state, even sleep is not restful.

It is a demonstration of the wonder of nature that a molecule like cortisol can have such wide ranging effects with normal blood levels of only 6 to 23 micrograms per deciliter.[8] In addition to the above mentioned effects, cortisol also plays a role in the body's carbohydrate metabolism, cardiovascular function, and inflammation. High levels of cortisol are known to cause weight gain, fatigue, and glucose intolerance. In the body no system stands alone. All parts are integrated and the action of one part will affect distant areas. In the production of ACTH, the pituitary does not act alone. It has to get its signal from somewhere, and that somewhere is the hypothalamus. This portion of the brain, along with the thalamus, is intimately associated with our emotional state. We can see why a disturbing event can cause our emotions to take over, as any emotional jolt sends a signal to the hypothalamus. It responds by increasing its production of cortiotropin releasing hormone (CRH). It is this chemical that makes its way to the pituitary, via the blood stream, to jar the gland into increasing production of ACTH. As ACTH is pumped into the blood, the adrenals kick into high gear leading to the symptoms of increasing anxiety, fear, and doubt. In addition, there is an increase in the blood pressure and the body begins breaking down glycogen, the storage form of glucose that is found in the liver. The body gets ready for flight, fight, or both. Do this enough times with the same stimulus and later watch as the body's physiologic and chemical memories cause the same physical symptoms to manifest, sans the threatening event. At this point the simple thought of an event is enough to rev things up and wear you out.

With all of the fluctuations that occur within our organism there has to be a chemical in the body that counteracts the effects of cortisol. The responsible agent is DHEA, or dehydroepiandrosterone. It acts as an anti-glucocorticoid (anti-cortisol). This drug is used by many patients suffering with HIV as an antidepressant, an energy booster, and for its muscle building capability as it is an intermediary in the pathway to the production of testosterone.[9]

A totally different chemical that helps keep balance in our body and mind is serotonin. This neurotransmitter's job is multifactorial, as it regulates our appetite, sleep patterns, mood, levels of aggression, and sexual behavior. Individuals going through major life changes and those unable to deal with unprocessed anger and aggression are prone to depression. One way to combat the debilitating effects of anxiety and depression is to raise the levels of serotonin in the synaptic junction. This space is where nerves communicate with each other. As a nerve impulse moves down an axon (nerve fiber conducting a stimulus away from the cell body of a neuron), serotonin is one of the many neurotransmitters that move across the gap to stimulate surrounding dendrites (nerve fibers that conduct a nerve impulse toward the cell body of a neuron). An axon can make connections with over 1,000 dendrites through synaptic junctions. The effects of not keeping serotonin in the synaptic junction are clearly demonstrated in those who suffer from anxiety and depression. Medications like Paxil, Effexor, Zoloft, and Lexapro, which are serotonin uptake inhibitors, allow serotonin to remain at the synapse for a longer period of time, thus the body relaxes and comes into balance under its influence.

In nature, the seed does not tell the soil what to feed it. The seed intrinsically knows what it has to accept from its surroundings. Why try to control the uncontrollable? Why spend so much time in worry and doubt when it adds nothing to achieving the desired outcome? It may be out of a false sense of power that we believe that worrying does any good at all. Worry is conditioned, and it kicks in when levels of cortisol bring you to a place where you no longer feel comfortable with what is in front of you.

If we get to the root of the learned response that initiated our tendency to worry and ruminate, then it becomes safe to drop the beliefs we have about worry. If we instead take that energy and constructively plan for what we want, then we can sit back and watch the expected changes come our way. When things do not turn out exactly the way we planned, we can be grateful for whatever comes our way, knowing that whatever it is, it will be right for us. Constantly running the same thoughts through our minds is a major waste of energy. You may ask: How do you let go of a thought? When you clench your fist, how do you make the tight, white knuckled hand release? You simply tell yourself that you are going to release the fist and the hand opens. What views do we hold that keep us from believing that we can't relax our minds and thus our muscles and attitudes? What makes you the victim of change instead of the originator of transformation?

Whether we want to believe it or not, all change depends on the choices we consciously or unconsciously make. Not everyone is equal in having the same variety of optimal choices as others, but we each have to do the best we can with what we are given. The more confidence we have in our problem solving skills, the easier it is to make the most appropriate choices. Myrna B. Shure, Ph.D., in *Raising a Thinking Child,* spells out and demonstrates the "I Can Problem Solve" Program. The perspective we take towards our problems and their solutions can be half the battle in bringing things to resolution. There are word pairs that we can play with that help us clarify our position on any issue. The word pairs that Shure uses as examples, and that are the most useful in her program, are the following: IS/IS NOT, AND/OR, SOME/ALL, BEFORE/AFTER, NOW/LATER, and SAME/DIFFERENT.[10]

When we are in the throes of change and experience uncomfortable levels of confusion, it is easy to forget to employ Shure's words. Instead, we find ourselves functioning on an all-or-none mentality, seeing everything as black or white, unintentionally ignoring the various shades and hues in between. Denial is a very powerful tool we use when the road ahead looks bleak and dark. As we rely more and more on denial, we find that the proposed and hoped for may be long in coming. Though *Raising a Thinking Child* was written as an instruction guide for parents who want to help their children learn the important art of critical thinking, more often than we would like to admit, we all act and think like children. This is especially so when we are stressed and in the middle of an ever-changing environment. It is not far-fetched to review some useful techniques to keep on the rim of consciousness so that they may be called upon the next time we are tested beyond our edge. Wrapped up in the multitude of everyday choices and having limited time to do what needs to be done, it is easy to lose sight of what is really happening.

Using the words IS/IS NOT helps us to reorient to the now. Relying on these words assists us in setting priorities and feeling comfortable with letting go of the less important concerns. IS/IS NOT analysis helps us deliberately define the boundaries of our problem. It helps us to focus on the correct issue as we commonly get off track when we are not in touch with our own boundaries. Possessing a muddy definition of the problem, we end up solving less important problems.[11] We have to constantly remind ourselves that what we think is important to us is not always a priority for those around us. When we happen to come upon a sensitive conversation, especially with a significant other or in a close work relationship, we can monitor our comments by first checking in with ourselves. By asking if our next thought IS or IS NOT helpful to the immediate situation, we exercise power over the encounter and have legitimate input concerning the direction and consequences of the encounter. If an accusatory or defensive thought is sparked and you are tempted to speak your mind, you have the power to diffuse or fuel the situation. If you know beforehand that the comment will raise defenses, it is worthwhile to check your thought and choose to listen more closely to what the other is saying. Taking a silent, calm, deep inhalation, and then calmly repeating what the other has said, in a show of understanding, will bring you closer together. By utilizing these two simple words, you can easily change how you interact with others and become more effective in your communication. You will also gain the respect of those around you.

In the center of uncertainty it, is natural to paint worse-case scenarios. By employing the IS/IS NOT test, we reorient and deal with real issues. The imaginary stuff lurking in our minds is allowed to fall by the wayside like yesterday's newspaper. Though you may think it is the end of the world if you do not make your next sale or if you don't win your next competition, the reality of the situation is that, in the process of coming to this point, you have learned many useful bits of information. Our minds have the capacity for unlimited creativity, so don't discard anything that you have worked so hard to achieve, even if the changes you have undergone to this point seem like a step backward. If you assume the attitude that nothing is ever wasted, you can walk away at the end of the day confident that you know more now than you did when you woke up. At this point you can ask: Is this something that I want to change, or shall I just watch events evolve as they will?

The next word pair, AND/OR, either helps us to broaden our choices, or they assist in helping us get more specific in what we want to see happen. If you are going to dinner and have concerns about your diet, you may choose to have soup AND salad, OR you may decide to have an entrée and skip dessert. You want to have an enjoyable time and you want to have a memorable dining experience, yet you want to take care of yourself and watch what you eat. How can you change how you view your diet and the image of yourself in the body that you have today? As you see yourself as a responsible adult - one who desires a healthier body and clearer mind - you can affirm this for yourself AND make your choices based on what is in keeping with your goal, OR you can succumb to your desire to fill yourself to the max and suffer the consequences of self-criticism after you have cleaned your plate. Just to entertain these thoughts the next time you go out, you are changing how you view your choices concerning your health, and in the process, you find you are taking more responsibility for the way you feel. Using the AND/OR technique gets you thinking critically.

In some situations it is possible to choose more than one option. Other times, it is practical to choose only one. A lot of this depends on how much effort it will take to achieve your goal. If you know that you have an hour to stop at the ATM, go to the dry cleaners, fill the car with gas, AND make a trip to the grocery store, OR continue surfing the internet, looking up the latest position of the Hubble telescope, and you know that later this afternoon you have to be one hundred miles away at a conference, your choices are limited and you will have to get done what needs to be done before your trip. On the other hand, if you knew that you would be free later in the day, then you could do both.

As an example of the subquery SOME/ALL, we can take a look at our work related responsibilities. To be ready for a presentation on Friday, you can do some work tonight and some tomorrow night, or you can watch TV and surf the net tonight, and stay up late tomorrow night and do ALL of the work then. In choosing to wait and do all of the work in one night, a pressure-cooker atmosphere may ensue. This may threaten your ability to use the same, critical thinking that would normally be exercised when the work is split up over two nights. In the rush to finish the project in one haste-filled night, the angst and the urgency to complete your task will spill over into the presentation the next day.

When we look at our options and know that we have a choice to get a project completed in one of the two manners listed above, then we can decide which way we would like to proceed. Knowing our own style, we give ourselves the benefit of having a greater chance of getting into the flow of the endeavourer. If we decide to rush the job and feel anxiety over our choice, then we know that next time we have the power to do things with the split schedule. It is a matter of paying attention to how you feel while doing your work and being willing to make your task easier the next time around. Things don't always have to be hard.

In order to view the consequences of our decisions, we can put the word pair BEFORE/AFTER to work. It is as if we now have the ability to have two perspectives on the subject and are able to alternate our view, reviewing things from these two vantage points. Our lives do not always proceed in a linear fashion, but the more points of references we have at our disposal, the more information we have at hand to take corrective action. When we realize that all of our choices have consequences, we can decide which path we want to take and recognize that, with all choice, there will be things that will have to be given up in order to gain in another area.

If you find that you are working too hard and feel that you would like to work less, then you will have to realize that when you worked full-time, there was more money to do some of the things that you wanted to do. Working at full and sometimes extra capacity, the limiting factor in doing what you want to do is the time element. In making a decision to go part-time, or to drop that second job, there will be more time to do things that you would never have fit into your schedule before you made the change. Balance is key, and in using BEFORE/AFTER, you will find this is a good tool to determine if your choice is a balanced one.

Albert Einstein once said, "The definition of insanity is when you keep doing the same thing and expecting a different result." When we frame the ideas SAME/DIFFERENT, we take advantage of categories that will allow us to further classify our thoughts, actions, and behaviors. How is it that, in the natural order of the universe, we persist in thinking that repetition of our same thought processes will lead to a desired end result, even when such a thought process failed in the past? What will it take to shift gears and say, "This is not working for me now, and what do I have to change to get what I want?" A particular behavior or belief may have worked for you in the past, but if you are no longer fed by that belief or behavior, then the only logical thing to do is to drop that belief and formulate a new one. How do we do that? By sitting quietly and viewing the movie screen of the mind; playing and replaying different scenarios until you find the one that fits best. This requires that you allow the old beliefs to drop. This is usually a most difficult thing to do, as we have grasping natures that make us feel uncomfortable when we try to let things go.

Frustration is an emotion we come up against every day. When we surrender our desire for change and remove our egos from telling us what we think we want, then we are free to tell ourselves that, even though we do not have what we want now, the possibility exists that it may come to us in the future. Taking this a step further, if we decide to be grateful for what we have now, then we can be confident that we will have what we need in the future.

Many times we are required to do what needs to be done in this moment and wait for a reward at a later time. Going to work, we know that in one to two weeks we will receive a paycheck. Your trust that the system is reliable is what keeps you going back to the job. If you found that after two weeks there was no check, your response of going to work would quickly extinguish. Bringing this idea closer to home, when we are thirsty we don't usually stop what we are doing and go for a drink immediately. Many times we put off our thirst and drink later, when the opportunity presents itself. We end up telling ourselves that we are busy and our thirst can wait. If we persist in putting off this need for fluids, we may one day find ourselves passing out and falling to the ground in a dehydrated state. Everything is measured in degrees, and sometimes changes happen so imperceptibly that we believe that there is an absence of change and that everything is stagnant. In retrospect, we find that nothing in this world is stagnant. Change is always happening.

Lacking any concept of patience, children want everything now. They interrupt family matters, butt in, and speak up, or blurt out their needs and desires without consideration for those around them. Early on, in an effort to keep the peace, parents drop what they are doing and meet the needs of the child. Eventually, with guidance and by example, the child learns to wait his turn and realizes that he is listened to with greater attention if he speaks in turn. With patience, we can begin to see the smallest signs of change and adjust to them on a daily basis, thus putting ourselves in a position to rarely be surprised at what happens.

What are you doing to meet your needs? How are you permitting the noisy inner voice to rule your days and get in the way of effective change? Are you not giving yourself any moments of solitude to create, dream, and focus your complete attention on those things that you need? The only way to complete any project or to meet a major goal is to bring together the fragments of moment-upon-moment thoughts where you can build one idea on top of the other. Then you can make adjustments and watch your desires manifest. Making uninterrupted time for yourself is critical so that you can sit and watch one coherent thought follow the next. As you pick out the patterns in your thoughts, the result is movement toward significant positive change.

Now you can make the decision to give yourself the gift of time so that later, as you learn more about yourself, you have more of yourself to share with others. Sometimes, just doing something with a minor twist or in a different order is enough to cause a major shift in the way you look at your world. It is all a matter of an inner energy shift. We get used to doing things one way, and until we question the validity of our choices, we will not make any changes. In *Your Handwriting Can Change Your Life*, Vimala Rodgers has taken the knowledge she has gained in graphology over the past thirty years and explains how our attitudes and self-concepts dictate what comes out on the written page. She, like many other writers, tells us that fear is what keeps us from expressing our hidden gifts and talents. In her short book, one that you can spend a lifetime in practice with, she takes the reader through her own alphabet: The Vimala Alphabet. Concerning her alphabet, she affirms the following:

> "Since each stroke of the pen reaffirms a thinking habit, and each thinking habit shapes our self-image, and self-image is the lens through which we see life, and this lens determines our behavior... if an alphabet were designed that exhibited only the most noble human traits, world peace might be a possibility."[12]

World peace may be a tall order, but we have to start with inner peace. In practicing our writing via the method of Rodgers, we find another avenue for self-exploration and positive change. In her writings, each letter of the alphabet falls into one of eight groups or families. Included in the Family of Communication are the following letters: A a, O o, D d, G g, Q q, and P p. These letters have to do with our ego and self-image, our verbal communication, our sensitivity, and our ability to draw personal boundaries. In addition, this family covers our beliefs about our prosperity and deserved praise, as well as our desire to serve humanity.

Another family division is that of the Family of Insight. This group includes letters that reflect innate spirituality, tolerance, perception, and intuition. The Family of Applied Creativity follows, and it includes the very important idea of balance in everything that we do. Other families relate to our capacity for flexibility and trust, our authority issues, and a separate family includes the letter Z alone, which represents where we stand in relation to perfect contentment.[13]

In a world of constant change, it feels good to have an influence over both the little and big changes that occur.

When we believe that what we wish to see happen will happen, we are brought into the creative realm. It may not be exactly the way we want it each time, but with trust, we find, we get what we need, and then some. We have the capacity to recreate ourselves, by choice, on a moment-upon-moment basis. This is a process that we can all learn to cultivate.

Notes: Changing Views

1. Information on the effect of hurricanes on the landscape can be found at *St. Petersburg Times Online*: "Growing Nature's Windbreak," at: http://www.sptimes.com/2005/07/23/Homes/Growing_nature_s_wind.shtml.

2. Ackerman, Diane, *An Alchemy of Mind*, (Scribner, New York, 2004), pp. 12-18.

3. Shreeve, James, "Beyond the Brain," *National Geographic*, March 2005, pp. 2-31.

4. Morrison, R, & O'Connor, RC, "Predicting Psychological Distress in College Students: The Role of Rumination and Stress," *Journal of Clinical Psychology*, 2004. http://www.stir.ac.uk/staff/psychology/ro2/JCP2004proofs.pdf. They site Martin, L.L. & Tesser, A (1996), "Some Ruminative Thoughts." In R. Wyer, Jr. (Ed.), *Ruminative Thoughts: Advances In Social Cognition*, Vol.11, (pp, 1-47). Hillsdale, NJ: Erlbaum.

5. For a through discussion on seed germination see: *Germination of Seeds*: http://users.rcn.com/jkimball.ma.ultranet/BiologyPages/G/Germination.html.

6. For further explanations and definitions of medical terms related to the pituitary gland and surrounding structures refer to *Medicine Net.com* @ http://medterms.com/script/main/art.asp?articlekey=9683

7. Dean, W, & English, J, *Hormone Salivary Testing: Key to Improving Hormone Balance*, http://www.vrp.com/art/469.asp

8. The normal cortisol level in the blood at 8 AM is 6 to 23 micrograms per deciliter. *Medline Plus*. http://www.nlm.nih.gov/medlineplus/ency/article/003693.htm

9. More on the hormonal effects in patients with HIV can be found in *New Theory on Body Fat Changes: Hormone Disruption by Protease Inhibitors May be the Root of Syndrome*. http://www.thebody.com/asp/mar00/lipodystrophy.html

10. Shure, M.B., & DiGeronimo, T.F, *Raising A Thinking Child: Help Your Young Child To Resolve Everyday Conflicts and get Along with Others: The "I Can Problem Solve" Program,* (Pocket Books, New York, 1994), pp. 11-39. 11. Further explanations on when to use and how to use IS/IS NOT analysis can be at Creating Minds.org. Web address: http://creatingminds.org/tools/is-is_not.htm#see

12. Rodgers, V, *Your Handwriting Can Change Your Life,* Simon & Schuster, New York, 2000), p.18.

13. Ibid, pp. 89-156.

CHAPTER 7

Who's in Charge: Authority Issues

In the days of lords and surfs, kings had the privilege of exercising ultimate authority. In a king's absence, the lord of the manner was charged with managing not only all of the land comprising the kingdom, but also its subjects. He yielded power over others with authority that encompassed decisions concerning life and death. In Avi's *Crispin: The Cross of Lead*, a children's book which earned the author the prestigious Newberry Medal, a boy of thirteen finds himself without parents.[1] For reasons unknown to Crispen, after his father died in battle, his mother, Asta, was shunned by the entire community. She and her son were poorer than the poorest poor of the village. Prior to his mother's death, the boy was only known and referred to as the son of Asta.

Only after his mother's death was it revealed to him by the bishop who befriended him, that his real name was Crispen. As another shock to the boy, on the same day that he learned his true identity, the lord of the manor proclaimed Crispen a "wolf's head". This meant that he could be killed, on site, by anyone. As he overheard this declaration while in hiding, he found himself on the run. Prior to being labeled a wolf's head, he had led a sheltered life, but through his efforts for survival, he began to interact and learn about his world. What he discovered was that he was actually the son of the deceased lord of the manor, which would have made Crispen the reigning lord. The current ruling party, in an attempt to maintain authority, was out to do him in. He was therefore charged with discovering his own authority, and he proceeded to do so though the use of his developing sense of power, fueled by each new encounter he faced.

In the days of Crispen, there was a need for organization, control, and management of the masses, and as we have seen, it was the king who had the final word on all issues. He had the power of life and death over all of his subjects. For the time it served humanity well, as keeping a community together so that resources could be pooled and unrest could be controlled was the only way for a society to remain coherent and have a chance to progress. In the days of Crispen, if you were walking in the woods and suddenly became hungry, it was not allowable to hunt for food; such an act - poaching on the King's property - could bring the death sentence. The only choice the common people had was to revolt and demand what they needed. In time, the unacceptable option of continued suffering under the reign of a harsh king was no longer palatable.

The church also had extreme power in formulating and maintaining rules for society. To settle personal disputes, bishops were given power to assign individuals to serve on *The Inquisition*. The most popular of these inquisitorial boards were in Italy and Spain. The number of lives ruined by the wishes and motivations of the select group of men in authority cannot be calculated. Over time, The Inquisition came to be feared by many because it had so much power. We, as a human race, still carry with us the imprint of the dealings our ancestors had with such a powerful entity. Much fear of authority has trickled down from days past, and whether good or bad, the original seeds of these fears have been long forgotten. No wonder we live with such anxiety today.

Imagine the feelings of helplessness that surfaced in the accused while standing in front of the stern, heavily robed, compassionless men in power. In a state of frenzy, fright, and despair, we can only imagine that their chests heaved, and every muscle fiber twitched, as their minds raced trying to find a way to avoid or change their upcoming fate. The myth remains today: when in front of The Inquisition, there is no future. Knowing that many were condemned to painful deaths, it is hard to imagine how anyone could be subjected to such conditions, stand there, and not break down. Many certainly did. Thinking beyond the victim, what were their survivors left with? The story of *Les Miserables* comes to mind where the well-known Jean Valjean served nineteen years in prison after stealing a loaf of bread to feed his starving sister's children. He was not intrinsically bad; he saw a need and did what he had to do to help. His options were to steal the bread or watch the children die of starvation. Would our actions be any different if we were in his situation?

The story of the French Revolution, 1789-1799, does not go as far back as Crispen's adventures, but during that time, people still lived under the rule of a monarchy.[2] Living under conditions where one person has absolute power over all undoubtedly breeds authority issues. It also breeds compliancy and conformity, unless one decides to rebel, in which case the price could be one's life. In the face of a rigid government that had no desire or motivation to have internal checks and balances, that had a growing bourgeoisie whose desire was to promote their own businesses, and that was entering into the Age of Enlightenment, where the ideas of ethics, aesthetics, and knowledge were becoming the motivating forces, the time was ripe for a revolution.

The Constitution of the United States tells us that we are all created equal; that no man should have power over another. If this is the case, why do so many individuals have problems with authority? When the idea of authority is entertained, images of the local or state police come to mind. They have the power to stop drivers and search cars as they work in their crisp uniforms, characteristic hats, set chins, and straight backs. Holstered guns and shiny black shoes offer a sizable degree of intimidation. Those who become police officers generally fit a certain personality profile. They are usually individuals who are not afraid of confrontation, have a high degree of self-confidence, and they are required to be physically fit, at least when they are first hired. They are trained to keep order, and know how to restore order when things are getting out of control.

In households, it is the older, bigger sibling who is put in charge. Responsibility is handed down from parents to the bigger child, and the little one becomes the subject of the ruling older. This only makes sense up to a certain age. Once the younger child is old enough to avoid injury, then the playing field should be leveled. It usually does not happen this way without a struggle, because the older sibling enjoys the power and is not willing to give it up. Many times, the younger individual gets so comfortable in the role of subservience that they never grow out of it to become an independent thinker. Sadly, they will always look to others to lead the way.

Controlling parents place their children at a disadvantage, because when it comes time for the youngsters to assert control and make their own decisions, they simply do not know how. This is so because they were never given the chance to practice. Anytime they attempted to exert authority they were put down and put back in their place in the family pecking order. Many parents fear giving up any control. This places children in a box and trains them in the ways of helplessness. As they grow into their futures, they succumb to the wishes and desires of others. They do not know how to ask for what they need because the needs of others always came first. They will do without and they will suffer because they were never given the chance to learn for themselves and taste their own power.

Zipping down the highway at seventy miles an hour in a fifty-five mile an hour zone, a sense of freedom fills the brain as the road ahead greets and invites us further along. With the radio on and the air conditioning chilling, we give thanks that we are able to experience a piece of heaven on earth. All of a sudden, an onward coming car flashes its high-beams and instinctively, we slow down. We know that a few miles ahead, there will be a state trooper grinning, his trigger finger on the radar gun, waiting to nab us, as we become one more number in a monthly quota of speeding tickets. As we heed the warning and take a slower pace, our eyes search for the sneaky officer ahead. For a moment we are compliant and cruise along, impersonating a law abiding citizen, but one to two miles down the road we pick up the pace and speed along like nothing happened.

At times like this, we know that we are doing what the law says is wrong, but we just don't care. We want to do what we want because it feels good. Besides, we're in a hurry and driving fast gets us to our destination quicker, so why slow down? Not to deny that there are concerns about getting caught, especially when thinking about the hefty fines and points levied by the insurance companies. There's a sinking feeling associated with paying extra on premiums, month after month, just because of one roadway indiscretion. But still, with boldness, we over ride the authority we know exists for the good of all.

Where did all of these notions come from? Of course, we picked up some of them from our parents, but we also formulated a number of them on our own because they appealed to us. With the stories we tell ourselves, there are certain images that blend and mix with what we believe. It's rewarding to make connections between reality and imagination. We allow ourselves to feel comforted in the middle of our incomplete knowledge by concocting images, real or not. The problems arise when we take these thoughts into the real world and speed to our destinations anyway. Not everyone is going to put themselves on the line for a little driving pleasure, especially at the risk of losing a driver's license, so some will follow the law to their best ability. For others, compliance will be so rigid that life turns miserable because of the internal stress generated in living up to societal expectations. There is a need to be obedient, especially in children, and as we grow older, desires may be put off at the cost of compliance—staying within the letter of the law, be it at home, work, or on the road. Unspoken law has become the authority and remains unrealized, thus when not allowed to proceed along the lines that you would like because of internal checks and regulations, a generalized sense of frustration arises. What's left is confusion.

Not only do we have the need for the approval of others, but a healthy emotional life also requires self-approval. If we fail to function in an approved manner, life will be fraught with anger. It can permeate our being and taint everything we do and say. We end up criticizing ourselves and others, and become locked in a state of paralysis. Our internal voice stops us from doing anything constructive, since we are defeated before we begin. We may stop in our tracks because of a lack of support due to the nature of the inner critic.

If you find yourself in such a position, it is necessary to keep moving forward, forging ahead, and doing what you believe is right for yourself, even in the face of a critic that is telling you that your efforts will not amount to anything. No voice can stop you unless you decide to appease it by doing what it says. Ignoring the critic just makes it stronger, as its voice gets louder and louder. One of the best tactics is to use the element of diversion and tell the critic to go do something that it enjoys on its own. Reassure the critic that it will be called upon when its powers of judgment and discernment are needed. When it is time to actually evaluate what you have chosen to do, the critic can serve you well. If what you have done in the past to silence the critic has not worked, then make the decision to try something different. Get creative by silencing your mind, quieting your breath, and listening to your inner guidance.

Stay in the flow for a while, even if you do not know where the process is taking you. It is all about trust, and as Bono tells us in his book, *Bono: In Conversation with Michka Assayas*, in every decision with which we are faced, our choices are always between trust and fear.[3] If you find that you have been living in fear, realize it is because you have chosen that path for whatever reason. The solution is to change your focus and keep your mind on trust. This too is a process, since building trust takes time, patience, and a willingness to move away from old ways of thinking. You know inside where you need to be, but in the past you relied on self-direction without the wisdom of experience, and self-doubt has kept you from moving forward. That is why your body is feeling tension and tightness. There has been too much need to control and too much trying to quell the inner harping of authority.

When you sit down with yourself in a moment of silence, whose voice do you hear? Is it your voice, and do you know what you sound like? Or is there incessant chatter in your head that is so loud that you can't make out what is being said over all of the internal confusion? If you do not hear your own voice, then it is time to figure out whose it is. Maybe it is the voice of your mother or father, or a teacher from the past. Maybe it is the voice of your boss, a spouse, or a co-worker. Maybe you listen to a trusted friend more than you listen to yourself. Once you determine who is in authority, ask yourself if you are comfortable with that voice, or if you feel that you are constantly nagged by its promptings. If you find that you are bothered by all of this, then begin digging for the reasons why you keep listening to this particular voice.

One of the first questions to ask yourself is: How do you get your own voice to take precedence over all other voices? In searching for your voice, it helps to begin writing and putting your ideas on paper. As you expose all of the real and imagined ideas of why you think you are the way you are, over time and with introspection, certain patterns will emerge. In the beginning of your writing, you may make many judgments, and this is natural and usual. Just keep writing and stay open to what comes up. At some point you will find what it is in your heart that is begging to be expressed. We all have a voice that speaks to us from our own inner wisdom. Trust that you will find it and you will.

In order to take a closer look at our inner workings and our relationship to authority, we have to ask ourselves the following: Who tells us what to do? From where do we get the words, thoughts, and ideas that move and motivate us? There is an origin to the signals that get us going and keep us going, and our job is to seek that place out and get to know the intricacies at play there. Deep below the surface of thought, below all the distractions, the wishes, and the perceived needs, there awaits the voice of wisdom. It is deep within the well, soft and quiet, ready to be heard only when everything else has been put aside. We have to be willing to drop our agendas and realize that the voice is trying to get us to listen. It may have been so weak and feeble in its attempts to make itself known, that maybe the voice has given up. If this is the case, there is reason for depression and despair. Any residual breath of life in the voice may just be hanging on, being squelched so many times it believes its own safety lies in continued silence. Maybe it is yelling, but your deaf ears will not let the sound in. The only way to reduce the screaming is to begin listening, no matter how loud, caustic, or accusatory the tone is. It is time to stop running away from your own wisdom. You know what you need, so start moving toward it in every way that you know how. Stop getting in your own way and listen to the one who knows.

Living like this is exhausting because it is a habit that is difficult to stop. It is time to brainstorm and figure out how to get the inner voice to speak for your needs. This is the path to the resolution of our self-induced suffering. Listen! Listen without judgment or reaction. Don't believe you already know what you are going to hear. Remaining open, you may hear something totally new. You will hear what you need to hear when you truly listen without inner comment.

As you listen, also feel. What does it feel like to just sit and listen? Do you find your patience getting short and your anger rising? Are there aspects of this impatience that frighten you or make you judge yourself or look to others to blame? There may be a feeling that you may never get over this deep-seated anger—that it will eventually consume you. You want to be rid of it, but have no idea how to do so. Even if you are feeling powerless over the presence of these recurring themes, still listen. Do not react or allow your mind to go off on a tangent of blame. Just listen. Quietly and gently listen. Listening like this may be the greatest gift you have allowed yourself to receive in quite a while. Be patient and open your senses, feeling what is present, but do not shut down. Without any desire to change or reject anything that comes up, listen.

If you are hearing words like "never," "forget it," "leave it alone," or "stop," then just keep listening. You are experiencing your resistance to listening. Go on… keep up the pace, hold on to what you set out to do, and listen. What authority figure is coming up? What is the need of the authority and how does it compare to your current needs and wants? Compare the two and see if there are any points in common. If there are major differences, it is up to you to decide where you will dedicate your time and energy. Take the positive input in common to both parties, and bring these needs into greater harmonic balance by weaving them into a common thread. Then, gently release the voice that is speaking to you as you weed out what you find is not in sync with your plan. With time and practice, new insight gained will find you thanking the authority figure for its input, then allowing it to go its own way. If fear arises and tells you that you can't do this on your own, remain focused on the common ground and look for even a glint of independence that you will allow to grow. This does not mean that you have to stand alone and be self sufficient from now on, but this new understanding is telling you that you are now capable of making your own decisions based on your needs and desires.

Much of what we understand of authority has been handed down from generation to generation through our dealings with the church and religion. For many, God is seen as the ultimate authority, but this should not allow any particular religious figure of today to claim that he or she knows what is best for you. People are looking for guidance wherever they can get it, and in today's world, the individuals with a solid platform and the power of charisma have the largest following. Such individuals should be viewed as instruments of the church, but not the ultimate authority. A painful example of a wolf leading sheep to slaughter involved Jim Jones and his followers at Jonestown, where because of his paranoia, Mr. Jones ordered over 900 of his followers, including 270 children, to drink cyanide-poisoned punch.

As mentioned above, the early courts of the church, whose members had authority over the people, were referred to as inquisitions. As far back as the sixth century, The Inquisition was viewed as an enemy of political liberty. Changes in Roman law around the First Century BC led to the development of this procedural process, but it wasn't until the thirteenth century that popes appointed individuals to function as an inquisitor. From 1478 on, a number of inquisitions were functioning in Spain, Portugal, Rome, and Venice. Most were abolished between 1798 and 1820.[4] The iniquity of The Inquisition lives in the minds of modern man to this day.

The problem then and now remains when an accuser makes an accusation out of malice. With early Roman criminal law, around the second century B.C., the accuser had to swear that he was telling the truth. We will always have the dilemma of trying to decide who is telling the truth and who is not, but the aspect of The Inquisition that continues to reside in our minds was the severe measures the Roman Catholic Church instituted to deal with those accused of failing to adhere to the doctrines of the church. Those who dissented, or deviated from the beliefs of the church, were tried under the rule of The Inquisition for heresy.

The word *heresy* derives from the Greek, *hairesis*, which around the first century, meant choice. By the fourth century, hairesis came to mean a difference between doctrine and belief.[5] If one chose to believe in ideas that were different from what the church taught, at first that individual would be viewed as needing teaching and conversion, but later such an individual would be burned at the stake.

When we look to others for leadership, we give away our authority and falsely tell ourselves that we do not know what is best for us. Failing to trust our inner knowledge, we give in to the words and recommendations of others, whereas to look at the big picture and take a chance at making the best decision for ourselves, our energies can be invested where they will be most effective for us. On the other hand, remaining ignorant of your own needs, you run the risk of persistent floundering like a bottom feeder. If you stand by and watch others getting what they want and settle for the minimum, you short-change yourself of joy, hope, and, trust. Not recognizing your own authority leaves the door open to the dangerous and toxic emotions of envy, jealousy, and greed. It is not too late to learn the right and proper way to take care of yourself and to recognize your own powers of authority over the direction of your life.

Is someone on your mind more than you would like to think is healthy? If you spend more time thinking about others and find that you are neglecting your own needs, it is time to consider ways of changing these thought processes and seek ways to fulfill your own needs. Many times we put others ahead of ourselves, thinking that they have figured out the meaning of life, and we look to them for external validation, not knowing how to get over our pain and move on with life. From this position of defeat, individual desire has been blotted out, and will remain so until acceptance of the pain and sorrow occurs. To fail to choose acceptance and recognize our own pain leaves the path to learned helplessness wide open.

In your own mind, who is calling the shots? Inquire to determine if you are still seeing events and experiences in your life through the eyes of a child and if you are making decisions based on circumstances from a time long ago. The chains of others are heavy and will bring you down until you realize that you are trying to meet the expectations of everyone except yourself.

A definition of authority from *The Concise Law Encyclopedia* tells us that authority is, in the broadest sense, just another way to explain permission. It is a right, coupled with the power to do an act, or order others to act. Of the various types of authority, "apparent authority" is expressed when a principal gives an agent various signs of authority to make others believe he or she has authority. This is the kind of authority that children deal with all of the time when it comes to interacting with their parents, family members, teachers and elders.

When we think about authority issues, teen-agers usually come to mind, as the teen-age years are those of spreading one's wings and budding independence. It is a time of experimentation and testing of limits. It is also a time of weighing the effects of peer pressure, and is only the beginning of dealing with authority issues. So, even if you are approaching middle age and feel you still have unresolved authority issues, it is time to give yourself a break. David M. Lawson explains, in *The Developmental Course of Personal Authority in the Family System,* that the majority of people who come to grips with family authority are between the ages of 30 and 45.[6] If we consider all of the psychological and emotional undertones of breaking away from the authority figures who paved the way to our future lives, it is not unexpected to feel overwhelmed.

The Theory of Personal Authority in the Family System (PAFS) was proposed by Williamson in 1991. PAFS is both an individual and family stage of adult development, with the task being "the renegotiation and termination of the hierarchical power boundary between the young adult and parents."[7] This is no small feat, as all of the decisions we make are grounded in what we have learned and received in terms of feedback or reinforcement, (good and bad) over the years. There will be conflict and the degree of difficulty will be determined by how open your parents were to incrementally giving up parental control along the way. If they were insecure and held on to their power, the task to autonomy is more difficult, and for some even impossible.

The unfortunate individual is the one whose parents were incapable of intimacy. Out of touch with their feelings, or because of past trauma or learned behavior, there was no way for them to open up and communicate effectively. In such families, members typically communicate only when they are annoyed with one other. There may be attempts at acts of caring, but even *they* fail to come off successfully because of ignorance over how to gracefully give or receive another's help in the face of dysfunction. In order to know another, there has to be some deeper understanding of your own inner workings. When families fail to show love and concern for each other, for whatever reason, then everyone suffers. It is only when the suffering becomes great that one of the members of the family asks themselves what is actually going on, and they begin the journey for the rest of the family - their intention being that they want to get to the bottom of things and find a better way for everyone to cope and prosper. The main problem associated with long-term, successful healing is the inability to deal with the pain that will inevitably follow, as it can be incredible and debilitating.

Intimacy has to do with trust, and if you do not trust yourself, you will look to others for direction and instruction. Once you find that you are not happy doing what you were led to do, intense anger surfaces. It is so powerful that you find it stressful to deal with. This leads to further frustration, and the cycle of anger and despair keeps you down-and-out.

Mikela Tarlow tells us about the power of intimacy in *Navigating the Future: A Personal Guide to Achieving Success in the New Millennium*. She explains that some of the obstacles to greater intimacy today are a result of our progress, as parents spend less than 8 minutes daily talking to their children. The average American watches six hours of television a day, and others spend countless hours on the internet.[8] Because of this, we are losing our connection with others, and with it, a chance for greater depth in our relationships. She continues to explain that in order to work successfully in our ever-changing, fast-paced world, where communication between managers and workers, and designers and consumers is getting tighter and more intense, we will have to know how to "get real."[9] We have to develop the skills to get to know who we are working with, and allow them to know us in order to work together effectively.

There has to be a point where we are willing to say that it is time to break down the walls that protect us. This also means that it is important to know the origin of your motivation, and that your drive comes from your own authority. We have to give ourselves permission to be the best that we can be, and not go around trying to please an inner critic or other co-dependent individuals.

One way that Tarlow tells us that we can "get real" is by emptying the space that we keep between us and other people. This space is made up of past projections that we have of others. By sticking with a past relationship, we find that it is the accumulated hurts, or supposed hurts, that are road-blocks toward greater intimacy. By dropping some of these feelings and working creatively to find new ways of relating, real connections can be established. There has to be a willingness to drop what you think you know and stay open to new interpretations. We can get real with ourselves by dropping ideas and concepts we developed years ago concerning who we thought we should be at a future time. It is when these previously made projections do not match with what is currently going on that disappointment sets in. This leaves us looking for someone else to blame, because the belief is that someone in authority is keeping our desired good from us.

If you find that you are letting past behaviors control how you relate to others, it is time to state your needs, face the unresolved conflicts, and start relating to others from a healthier vantage point, with the understanding that no one person should have control over another. If you have lived a life in any one of the following modes, then there is work to be done: living by the means of over-functioning, under-functioning, fighting, pursuing, or distancing that has kept you from individual and/or social intimacy. If you are fed up with the person you were years ago, it is time to ask: Why keep on living the life of one who is asleep? There does not have to be a rude awakening, but there has to be some prodding to get the mind thinking in a new way—a way that is separate from past restrictions that were based on fear motivated behaviors.

As Harriet Lerner, Ph.D. tells us in *The Dance of Intimacy*, "We move up on the selfhood scale (and the intimacy scale, for that matter) when we are able to:

- Present a balanced picture of both our strengths and our vulnerabilities.
- Make clear statements of our beliefs, values and priorities, and then keep our behavior congruent with these.
- Stay emotionally connected to significant others even when things get pretty intense.
- Address difficult and painful issues and take a position on matters important to us.
- State our differences and allow others to do the same."[10]

When we fail to do the above, we set ourselves up for manipulation and open ourselves to the beck-and-call of others. Instead of falling back on the old ways of isolating ourselves from conflict, even though it puts us right in the middle of our anxiety, it is possible to work through the difficult feelings and come to higher ground. Taking a stand and committing ourselves to the idea that we will begin to look at our pain no matter what comes up, we find that fear is truly a state of mind, and it doesn't have to be our reality. Instead of focusing on what we know our weaknesses to be, it is healthy to look at our strengths. The issue becomes one of how we view our strengths. If we think that kindness toward others is a weakness, then it is necessary to challenge this incorrect thinking pattern and realize that kindness is a sign of strength.

We can take our talent for persistence and apply it to changing the way we look at authority. The goal becomes one of giving ourselves permission to do what we think and feel will bring us fulfillment—things that will feed and nurture us. Marcus Buckingham & Donald Clifton explain to readers that even a perceived negative trait, such as dyslexia, can be used as a talent as long as you can find a way to use it in a productive way. They tell the story of David Boies, a United States government lawyer. He is dyslexic, yet was able to deliberately and politely frazzle Bill Gates in the government's antitrust suit against Microsoft. He consciously stays away from fancy, high-sounding words for fear of tripping up on them, but he comes across clearly using simple, easy to understand words.[11]

There are specific ways to begin honing in on our individual talents. Buckingham and Clifton encourage us to pay attention to our first reactions to the events that occur around us. In a crisis situation, you may find your usual response is to take responsibility and try to diffuse the charge, or make a humorous comment to relieve the pressure, or inquire about another's misfortune to change the focus, or seek out minute details in an attempt to dissect the situation. Patterns of thinking and acting emerge as we pay attention to our first thoughts. Getting into the habit of monitoring these thoughts, we gain a better idea of the way we routinely respond in uncomfortable times. Knowing ourselves better leads to greater confidence in our chosen path, and we are less likely to have authority issues, as we tell ourselves that it is acceptable, and even preferable, to be the way we are.

Other cues to pay attention to in order to identify our strengths are yearnings, rapid learning, and satisfactions.[12] When you take the time to step back and ask yourself what you are drawn to, you find that the thought or image has been recurrent over time. You may have put off following an interest because of concerns of the day, like paying the rent, mortgage, electric bill, or car payment. With everything you need to do, it seems impossible to find the time to pursue your desire. By taking these yearnings seriously and trusting that what you dwell on will manifest, the path ahead will clear, leaving more time and energy for the endeavor that is calling you. It is a matter of recognizing your priorities and acting on the information. Ask yourself what the next step is in the fulfillment of this desire, and follow through, even though you have no idea what will happen next.

If you find that you have acquired a new skill with a fair amount of ease, then this may be a sign that your talent is at hand. If you have been waiting for permission to move ahead in this new endeavor and find you are stalled, it is imperative that you take a hard look at what exactly it is, or who it is, that is holding you back. If a vision of a family member comes to mind, see what it is about your relationship that you have been upholding to keep the peace. Then see what you can do to bring the relationship toward greater balance. If you fear moving ahead or becoming successful in a new venture because you believe it would upset a significant other, identify that as an obstacle to be overcome. Look ahead, see yourself doing what you want to do, and take the steps to make it a reality. As you begin and find you are taking heat from another for the changes you are undergoing, turn your attention to inquiring what it is they would like to pursue and encourage them to do so. Try to move ahead together, dropping all notions of competition, and seek creative solutions to the challenges ahead. We all have gifts, but many times we fail to take the opportunity to discover just what they are.

If you feel it is a significant other that is "holding you back", be honest with yourself and inquire if you are using this person as an excuse not to act. Maybe staying where you are and not risking failure feels safer than going out into the unknown. You may fear that you will not like the new you, and will be stuck with a new set of rules after doing all of the work required for your desired result. It is beneficial to put your thoughts out in the open so those close to you know what it is that you are expecting. The act of verbalizing, in the form of telling another what it is that you want to do, will force you to take a look at the real possibility of it happening. This may be one reason why you are not open concerning your desires, because deep down you know you have not done the preliminary work in arranging things for a successful outcome. Your partner will hopefully call you on your plans, and until you have a fairly clear picture of where it is that you want to go, there will be holes to fill. If you are lucky and have a supportive partner, he or she will help you fill in the blanks. The reality of the situation is that you have the final word in everything that you chose to do or not do.

Melody Beattie offers us good advice in her book, *Codependent No More,* when she advises us to live our own lives.[13] If we are so concerned with what other people think, then we will continually be influenced by these thoughts, and everything we attempt will be colored by our perceived concepts of what the other wants us to do. It is one thing to show concern for others, yet it is detrimental to your mental and physical health to be overly consumed by pleasing others. Ms. Beattie tells us that it is necessary to detach ourselves from others. In saying this, she does not imply that we disconnect from others and live a life of isolation, but she is suggesting that we stop blaming others for our misfortunes and take responsibility for our lives. We have to find a way to get comfortable with all of our fears, doubts, and faults.

By dropping all of the "shoulds," and letting go of the need to please, we allow ourselves to release the wish to meet everyone's needs. Then, space and time will open up to find the things that you enjoy. When it comes to who should be the authority in your life, the revelation that you are the responsible one is life-changing. Once you truly grasp this concept, it becomes easy to take care of yourself. As you begin doing what needs to be done for your best health and interest, then you will find doors opening that allow you to begin to fulfill your higher purpose. As Bettie says, "Self-care is an attitude of mutual respect. It means learning to live our lives responsibly. It means allowing others to live their lives as they choose, as long as they don't interfere with our decisions to live as we choose. Taking care of ourselves is an art, and this art involves one fundamental idea that is foreign to many: giving ourselves what we need."[14]

Notes: Who's in Charge? Authority Issues

1. Avi, *Crispen: The Cross of Lead* (New York, Scholastic, 2002).

2. More information on the French Revolution and the events surrounding it can be found at: http://en.wikipedia.org/wiki/the_enlightenment.

3. *Bono: In Conversation with Mitchka Assayas* (New York, Riverhead Books, 2005).

4. Edward Peters, *Inquisition* (Berkeley and Los Angeles, University of California Press, 1989), p. 1-10.

5. Ibid. p.19.

6. Lawson, D.M., & Brossart, D. (2004). "The Developmental Course of Personal Authority in the Family System." *Family Process,* 43, 391-409.

7. Williamson, D.S. *The Intimacy Paradox: Personal Authority in the Family System.* (New York, Gilford Press, 1991).

8. Tarlow, M. *Navigating the Future: A Personal Guide to Achieving Success in the New Millennium.* (New York, McGraw Hill, 1999), p. 193.

9. Ibid. p. 197.

10. Lerner, Harriet. *The Dance of Intimacy: A Woman's Guide to Courageous Acts of Change in Key Relationships.* (New York, Harper Perennial, 1989). p. 35.

11. Buckingham, M., & Clifton, D.O. Now, Discover Your Strengths. (New York, Free Press, 2001), pp. 48-61.

12. Ibid. pp. 67-75.

13. Beattie, Melody. *Codependent No More: How to Stop Controlling Others and Start Caring for Yourself.* (San Francisco, Harper Collins, 1987), pp. 113-118.

14. Ibid. p. 115.

CHAPTER 8

The Art of Doing Nothing

It's the top of the ninth, bases are loaded, the count is three balls and two strikes, and the crowd is standing, anticipating the next pitch. The score: 0-0. Anyone not versed in the ways of baseball would think that nothing has really happened during this most recent outing of highly paid, grown men playing on a grassy field. It's as plain as day by the scoreboard that no team has had a single run. Those who follow the game know that the numbers below the actual runs per inning have significance also. In this game each team has six hits and two errors, yet the score remains 0-0. All four errors were whoppers, and each one of them will be replayed on the sports news tonight for all sports fans to see. All of the mistakes are enough to get a die hard fan down. A cause of a deep depression it's not, but maybe a mild case of the blues for the rest of the evening.

Let's turn our attention to individuals living through serious bouts of depression. On the surface it would appear that they are listless and lethargic, spending most of their time on the sofa or even in bed. They go to bed early and wake up late. Their movements and speech are slow. They think slower than usual. In The Zen Path through Depression, Philip Martin tells us, "The gray place, that depression is can be frightening and disorienting. Whether or not you have been there before, each time is different...Stumbling in fear and panic, we become more lost. In depression, we often run until we become swallowed up in the darkness that has become our life." It is Mr. Martin's next phrase that is the point of focus for this chapter. He tells us, "What may be crucial to our healing is, first, to do nothing." [1]

You read this and the objections arise: "How does he expect me to just sit around and do nothing? I have so much to do in the next twenty minutes - *you* pick the chore: feed the cat, go to the store, visit my mother, dress the kids, finish this report, trim the bushes, get some sleep. Although I would love to sit around and do nothing, I just don't have the time." In today's high-tech environment, "big brother" has a good idea of what Americans do with their time. The second annual release of the American Time Use Survey (ATUS), sponsored by the Bureau of Labor Statistics, and conducted by the U.S. Census Bureau focuses on the time Americans worked, did household activities, cared for household children, and participated in leisure and sports activities in 2004. [2]

On an average day in 2004, persons in the U.S. aged 15 and above slept over 8.5 hours, had over 5 hours of leisure and sports time, worked for 3.7 hours, and were busy doing household chores for 1.8 hours. The remaining 4 to 5 hours were spent eating and drinking, attending school, and shopping. Persons who were employed full-time worked 9.2 hours on weekdays, spent 7.5 hours sleeping, had 3 hours for leisure time, and either had unkempt, dust bunny-filled, or extremely small houses, as they spent only 0.9 hours doing household activities. [3]

The ATUS data has has just recently been updated, and unfortunately the average American is spending more time than ever watching television. More Americans are working less hours on weekends and are spending the extra time on leisure activities and sleep. Leisure activity included watching TV, socializing, and exercising. In the most recent report, a gender gap has developed over leisure time, as women are spending 5 fewer hours per week on leisure time than men. This tells us that women are working more hours on the job, and have not cut back on housework. [4]

The picture gets a bit more stifled when we consider households with children. In families where the youngest child is under 6, time spent providing care averaged 2.7 hours for women, and 1.2 hours for men. Physical care, playing with children, and travel related to childcare took up most of the time spent in childcare activities. Even so, adults living in households with a child under age 6 spent 4 hours a day doing leisure and sports activities. [5]

In the ATUS survey, watching TV was the leisure time activity that occupied the most time, as it comprised half of the leisure time activity for both men and women. The next most common leisure time activity was socializing, which accounted for 45 minutes per day for both sexes.[6]

We all know that most of us spend way too much time staring at the TV, and for those with cutting-edge technology, it must be more difficult to pull away from the brighter-than-life pictures displayed in all their glory. In the survey, there is no mention of how many folks just sit around and do nothing. We seem to lack the courage and desire to consciously take time away from the call of the day to just sit with ourselves in silence. We all seem to be living as if it is dangerous to be idle. Reading this, you may think of doing nothing as equivalent to idleness. Bible readers will be quick to tell us that 2 Thessalonians 3:6 contains a warning against idleness as it admonishes us to, "keep away from every brother who is idle and does not live according to the teaching you received from us."[7]

This discussion on the subject of doing nothing is far removed from the concepts of idleness, self-indulgence, slothfulness, or anything to do with being a sluggard. It has nothing to do with being lazy or dodging one's work. In fact, to truly do nothing takes a great deal of effort, as the mind just wants to go everywhere and be in all places at once. Here, doing nothing is a different way of suggesting that we need to spend more time being present. Doing nothing, in the figurative sense, creates space that allows us to drop past concerns, and prevents us from jumping ahead to future potential roadblocks. B.K.S. Iyengar, the yoga master who brought the practice to the west over 50 years ago, cautions us that *savasana* (the pose where we imitate a corpse and lie perfectly still) is one of the most difficult in yoga because it is much harder to keep the mind still than it is the body.[8]

What we are seeking in our time of doing nothing is our center. We all need to ground and know in our hearts that we are just a small part of a temporary, living planet. Our choices, actions, and reactions affect those in our circles, yet too many times we make decisions based on the expectations of others. We say "yes" when we want to say "no," many times out of the fear of consequences, and other times to avoid confrontation. In living from our center, there is a greater probability of expressing genuine action, and thus less room for conflict or struggle.

Thomas Edison, the ubiquitously known inventor of the light bulb, became totally deaf in his left ear and lost 80% of his hearing capacity in his right ear. Apparently, he was born with a partial hearing deficit and became almost totally deaf either from a blow to the head by a train conductor, or as a result of scarlet fever when he was fourteen years old. He adapted by using the silence to sharpen his powers of concentration. Later, when he would have been able to have an operation to restore his hearing, he refused on the grounds that in the noisy world around him, he would find it difficult to re-channel his thinking.[9] His deafness created a void for him that allowed him to think in much different ways than his peers.

Another story of creativity and innovation employing our deeper mind comes from Madhukar Shukla in his description of the discovery of the chemical structure of benzene. August Kekule was trying to figure out the structure of this organic compound when he fell into a dream state. He described the following to a group of scientists explaining the process:

"... I turned my chair toward the fireplace and sank into a doze. Again the atoms were flitting before my eyes. Smaller groups now kept modestly in the background. My mind's eye sharpened by repeated visions of a similar sort, now distinguished larger structures of varying forms. Long rows frequently rose together, all in movement, winding and turning like serpents; and see! what was that? One of the serpents seized its own tail and the form whirled mockingly before my eyes. I came awake like a flash of lightning. I spent the remainder of the night working out the consequences of the hypothesis." [10]

Benzene is a chemical solvent. Since it possesses an odor, it is referred to as an *aromatic* compound. It forms the basic framework for other chemicals with which we are all familiar, such as toluene, TNT, and even aspirin. Benzene was originally discovered by Michael Faraday in 1825, but it wasn't until 1858 that Kekule was able to determine its chemical structure. In "sleeptalk" terms, when Kekule saw the vision of the energetic serpent, he was in a state of *hypnagogic* sleep. There are states of hypnagogic, or sleep paralysis, where one is unable to move or talk for about one minute when falling asleep. In addition, there can be visions that are referred to as "hypngogic hallucinations", with vivid, usually terrifying dreams and sounds, but Kekule was probably in a simple form of hypnagogic sleep. This state differs from *REM* sleep (the rapid eye movement state that we experience during dreaming, where our bodies are paralyzed at the level of the brain, so that we do not act out our dreams) in that during the hypnagogic state, the sensory cortex may be receiving both externally and internally generated information.[11]

So even during sleep, there is a lot more going on than we think. Besides the 5 stages of sleep, (stages 1-4, followed by a period of REM sleep) there are sub-states of sleep, such as those referred to previously. The deepest state of sleep is experienced in stage 4, when electromyograms that measure brainwave activity show slow wave, or *delta wave* sleep. In this state there is very little eye movement, muscle activity is minimal, and if awakened from this stage, we find ourselves groggy and disoriented.[12] It is in this stage of sleep where we are probably closest to a state of nothingness. The only caveat here is that it is in Stage 4 sleep, sleepwalking and sleeptalking are are most likely to occur.[13] It is somewhat paradoxical that we are capable of walking and talking in our sleep when brain activity is at its lowest, but such is the wonder of the mind.

Zero is typically equated with nothingness. It is the absence of everything, similar to the conditions we would expect to find in a vacuum. The thought-energy and mathematical formulations applied in efforts to understand the nature of a vacuum are beyond the comprehension of all but those who study physics and mathematics as their life's work. For a taste of the complexity involved in explaining the state of a vacuum, I refer you to an article titled *The Physics of the Vacuum*.[14] In it you will find phrases such as the following: the vector potential wave equation, zero point energy, oscillator energy, fermion energy, negative energy states, eigenvalues, annihilation and creation operators, bosons, and the uncertainty principle.

This is all very complex information, but some of the concepts are familiar to all of us. For example, the *vector potential wave equation* refers to something in physics known as the "Aharonov-Bohm effect". It tells us that potentials (charged particles) that pass close to, but do not encounter a magnetic or electrical field, will change their dynamics in subtle yet measurable ways.[15] This is similar to what ethologists were telling us years ago in that when we study the behavior of an animal, we change its behavior. All of this reflects back to the idea that everything in our universe is inter-connected, and there is no getting away from this fact.

When we work to remain isolated and protected in self-made vacuums, dysfunction and malfunction prevail. Our interpretation of events can lead us to build walls that keep us from experiencing life fully. As inner tensions build up, they are supported by an ever- hardening outer façade, and as we persist in telling ourselves that the words and actions of others do not bother us, we effectively condition ourselves to ignore our feelings. Unable to deal with painful emotions, we do not realize the fact that we are deeply hurt by what we perceive is happening.

As we all know but fail to remember: Nothing in life occurs in a vacuum. We believe our behavior does not affect those around us and go about our business thinking only about "numero uno." We need to take care of ourselves in the proper way, but think how much more fulfilling life would be if we break down the walls of isolation and ever more frequently stay truly open to the ideas and concepts of those around us. Such sharing brings us all toward common ground and helps to break the cycle of worn-out, repetitive thought patterns.

Going a little deeper into the science mentioned above, an *eigenvalue* tells us the sum of a combination of vectors in physics and mathematics. *Vectors* have to do with the direction an object takes. We have our own vectors, or directions in life, and keeping with the law of averages, we are happy with some of the directions and not so satisfied with others. As long as the sum of these vectors is in a positive direction, then overall, we sail along with a general tendency toward being satisfied with life. On the other hand, if we train ourselves to think independently of the direction of our vectors, then we open ourselves up to experience greater joy. We can know contentment, and maybe even happiness, despite any and all negativity that may be going on around us. In this scenario contentment is assured.

Other technical uses for eigenvalues and eigenvectors are to compute stability analysis, the physics of rotating bodies, and small oscillations of vibrating systems.[16] We are all vibrating bodies, but as we age every part of our bodies begin to desiccate and tighten up. A perfect example is in the case of back pain. The disc that acts as a cushion between each of our vertebral bones in our back, the *nucleus propulsus*, with incorrect use will slip out of its normal anatomical position. Sciatica occurs when a disc is forced out of place, usually from lifting or bending in a manner that does not support the lower back. As we get older, these discs desiccate and shrink, thus making them more likely to dislocate when stressed. To intentionally keep these parts of our bodies vibrating and functioning optimally requires thoughtful action every day of our lives. Continuing to push on with your usual activities while your nervous system is sending you signals in the form of pain impulses will lead to damage of tissues and eventually, chronic pain. It is far wiser to stop what you are doing, reassess the situation, and take appropriate action that will still allow you to continue in your activity, but without the strain and pain.

Another example of our vibrating natures is seen when we attempt to lift an object that is heavier than we are capable of lifting. Our muscles twitch and shake under the strain. The shakes and tremors are the muscle's way of trying to wake up and go to work for us, but if they are lazy from disuse, they will complain long after the lift. Here again, it is better to stop what you are doing (do nothing), lighten the load, or call for assistance.

Taking one more look at eigenvalues and eigenvectors: they help mathematicians solve problems in linear transformation (changes occurring in a uniform manner) by pairing each linear transformation with its corresponding matrix. A *matrix* is a mathematical device used to solve problems that depend on two categories. Converting a matrix into a diagonal matrix provides a way to bring a system into the simplest possible form. In mathematical terms, a diagonal matrix reduces the number of parameters from $n \times n$ for an arbitrary matrix, to n for a diagonal matrix, and thus the characteristic properties of the initial matrix can be determined.[17]

It is this simplest form possible that we are seeking when we dwell on the idea of doing nothing. It is a healthy place to reside when we go about our business and not add the unreal, extraneous stuff fabricated by our minds. In looking to do nothing, it is necessary to consciously not add anything else to what we are seeing, feeling, or thinking. We are looking for a pure state: one of raw consciousness, accepting what is, without judgment or criticism.

From the above, we see how complex it is to bring a concept to its simplest form. Every day, on the radio and in magazines, we read how we should live more simply. We are encouraged not to shop to the point of debt, and are told to resist impulse-shopping and credit purchases, where the burden of payments may extend half-way into the next year. We are not comfortable with the idea of nothing. In fact, many times when we listen to the success stories of others, we hear that some significant other in their past told them that they we would never amount to anything. Paradoxically, such images present a challenge, and many times become the seeds for success.

We can get comfortable with the idea of doing nothing, but in order to do so, we have to drop all ideas of where our eigenvectors are taking us. The ancient Greeks were so uncomfortable with the concept of zero that they never introduced a symbol for zero.[18] When we review the Roman numerals, we also find, there is no zero. Even as far back as 3000 BC, the Egyptian hieroglyphic system had no need for a symbol meaning zero. Their system is an early example of a decimal system, having symbols for numbers that carry no positional information, thus there is no need for a zero.[19] The Babylonians were the first to introduce a symbolic representation of zero, but it was never meant to be used as an endpoint where nothing was to remain. It was simply used to distinguish an empty space in an accounting register.[20]

All of this talk of higher math and ancient accounting systems is not meant to take us away from the realities of our daily grind, but is presented as a metaphor for our innate resistance to the concept of conscious nothingness. On the grassroots level, when we talk about doing nothing, I am referring to using the moments when we are stunned and blank from overwork, excess, or exhaustion. It is at these times, when we have no other option but to give up our struggles, that we begin to pay attention to our surroundings and acknowledge where we are, even if only by default.

Most of us are fearful of insomnia. Knowing that the coming day has unforeseen challenges, we want to be at optimal performance, working effectively and enjoying what we are called to do. As we lie awake at night with our eyes open, the reality of the stationary ceiling fan over our head, made visible by the nightlight in the hallway, brings us back into the room. We have moved from the unreal images of the imagination to the real. We are now looking at what is right in front of us, and it is refreshing. Doing nothing, in this situation, is more productive and pleasing than wallowing away the time in a runaway imagination that is filled with worst-case scenarios.

Our brain's video may have been rehashing a troublesome experience or projecting us into an uncertain future, leaving us in a deeper state of anxiety. Dwelling on a previous hurt of which we have not yet learned to let go, we end up wallowing in a sticky quagmire of dark emotions. With feelings too thick to penetrate, the sense of being overwhelmed keeps us imprisoned. If we are lucky, and if we have been working toward the goal of being more present, we find ourselves thankful for the fan in the room. It was the instrument that brought us back. No longer in the mind-zone, we become aware of our partner's sleepy breathing as they continue to rest. If we are even luckier, we begin to get the idea that right now we are doing nothing. Sure, we are seeing and hearing, but we are not actively engaged in trying to work anything out. Our plans and scheming natures are put on hold, and that offers relief.

If we go with it and continue to observe, and see how the light bends across the ceiling, and how the shadows intersect with the corners of the room, we might begin to feel. First, we feel our backs against the mattress, supporting our strained and battered bodies. As we take note of this, the muscles naturally lengthen and begin to respond to our breathing. We may have images of past relationships as the muscles shift. If we do not scare ourselves or allow ourselves to go down the path of blame and anger, we might begin to experience the warmth of forgiveness. All of this happens when we allow ourselves to do nothing. In a moment, the heat kicks on in the room. The shade gently and rhythmically taps against the door as it is nudged from stillness by the moving air. The tapping is in rhythm with the heartbeat.

How exactly does all of this happen? It happens through grace. The greatest obstacle to receiving grace is pride. According to Philip Yancey, author of *What's So Amazing About Grace?*, "Grace is Christianity's best gift to the world, a spiritual nova in our midst exerting a force stronger than vengeance, stronger than racism, stronger than hate.[21] We all know the word *grace*. Some of us say grace before each meal, or at least before the evening meal, but how many of us live in grace? How many of us have ever taken the time to even think about what this means? This is a concept that takes some thought.

According to the Merriam-Webster Online Dictionary, the word grace ultimately finds its roots in the Latin gratia, meaning favor, charm, or thanks, and from gratus, meaning pleasing or grateful. It is the "unmerited divine assistance given humans for their regeneration or sanctification."[22] The difficulty in understanding this term stems from our ingrained social order, which tells us that we are to be recognized by our works, by what we do, and by what we accomplish. When it comes to receiving grace, all that is required is that we accept it.

As noted in a June 2004 Fox News Poll, 92% of Americans said that they believe in God.[23] This high percentage of belief has persisted since the Gallup Poll started asking Americans whether they "believe in God or a universal spirit" in 1944. These percentages are in sharp contrast to the numbers obtained in 1991 and 1993 by the International Social Survey Program (ISSP), which surveyed individuals in seventeen countries worldwide. Some of the representative countries included the United States, Northern Ireland, the Philippines, Italy, Great Britain, Russia, Hungary, and others. In the ISSP poll, less than 63% of those questioned reported that they believe in God. It is felt that the ISSP responses required a degree of certainty that is not present in the Gallup Poll, and brings to question the conviction Americans have in their belief in God.[24]

In order to know grace, we have to put aside our will, stop trying to calculate the best way to make our dreams come true, and just appreciate the gift of the incoming breath that is giving us life. If the quoted numbers above can be relied upon, and anywhere from 60-90% of the world population believes that there is a God or some other higher power, then why are we not all living in the light of grace? Why do we continue struggling to make our way in the world?

Charles R. Swindoll, in *Paul: A Man of Grace and Grit,* has made an extensive study of the life of the apostle Paul. In addition to growing up in a city rich with cultural and commercial diversity, Saul (Paul's name prior to finding Christ) was "the beneficiary of an equally rich religious and intellectual heritage."[25] As Swindoll tells the story, Saul couldn't wait for the day when he would become a member of the Jewish Supreme Court, the *Sanhedrin*. He was a successful lawyer whose abilities were far beyond those of his contemporaries. With the rise in Christianity, the ruling religious leaders feared for their positions of power. Saul also felt that he needed to squelch the activities of the Disciples of Christ. Swindoll describes Saul's state of mind in the following passage:

"Saul's blood is boiling. He's on a murderous rampage toward Damascus. He charged north out of Jerusalem with the fury of Alexander the Great sweeping across Persia, and the determined resolve of William Tecumseh Sherman in his scorching march across Georgia. Saul was borderline out of control. His fury had intensified almost to the point of no return. Such bloodthirsty determination and blind hatred for the followers of Christ drove him hard toward his distant destination: Damascus. If you were a follower of Jesus living anywhere near Jerusalem, you wouldn't want to hear Saul's knock at you door".[26]

It was on the road to Damascus where Saul was struck blind by God's intervention. Prior to this, Saul believed that he was persecuting followers of a false Messiah, but after being touched by God he became not only blind, but confused and bewildered. Once his sight was returned, he retreated to the Arabian Desert where he spent a thousand plus days alone.[27] It was there, in the barren solitude, in a place where he could do nothing but think, where he developed a deeper understanding of the grace of God.

We all want things. Look at all of the advertising that engulfs us. On television, we have the shopping networks flashing their wares twenty-four hours a day. There is the internet with its pop-ups, telling us we have won the newest audio or video device. All that we have to do to win is to buy so many items within a certain time period. Daily, we are tempted to buy a new car by constant bargain offerings, and we are told that our living space is never big enough or convenient enough by today's standards. No wonder credit card debt is at an all time high.

We want all of this stuff and are willing to go into debt to get some of it, but we are blind to accepting the free gifts that are ours for the taking. It doesn't cost us anything to look into the eyes of our children when they speak to us. We are not billed if we sit and listen to our five-year-old son or daughter as they tell us a twenty-minute story about the pictures they drew while we were at work. We think we will lose something - maybe our edge - if we are not constantly thinking about ways to get ahead or keep up, but if we fail to receive the free gifts we are given, we find we are the losers.

Grace is free. We do not have to do anything to earn it. As a doctor I do not have to see thirty patients a day to feel that I have earned the love of my family or the love of my patients.

There is no figuring anything out. No effort, toil, or sweat is necessary. There are no deadlines or clocks when it comes to accepting grace. All that is required is a willingness to receive it. Like everything else, there are conditions that have to be met to receive this gift. We have to be willing to give up control, willing to be present, willing to drop all thoughts of blame, fear, and doubt. We have to stand at the door and open it.

My prior work took me to a satellite office forty miles from home, every third week, to see patients. About every six weeks I was fortunate enough to see a gentle, kind, elderly lady who I had treated for multiple myeloma. Thanks to newer treatments, her disease was well under control. She was a widow and lived alone in a big house in town. Her greatest challenge was the indolent, yet progressive onset of dementia that had insidiously developed over a year or two. Thanks to the pharmaceutical industry and its research efforts, with the use of medication, she was able to remain self-sufficient and was not a danger to herself or others.

On her visits she would tell me how things were with her. She shared her health concerns and described how she occupied her time. She appreciated the health that she had and watched her blood sugar, though not to the point of obsession. As she spoke, it was without pretense. There were no ulterior motives behind her words. She simply wanted to talk and connect with another human being. Her gifts to me were her honesty and sincerity, and the pleasure she seemed to experience as she shared her stories with me for those ten minutes every six weeks.

Through grace, she remained independent and was able to walk and speak with integrity. As much as possible for her condition, she knew herself, and that was admirable. For me to experience her offerings, all that was necessary was to just sit and listen. If I worried about how many more patients I had to see or who I had to call next, I would have thrown away an opportunity to experience a real connection and a true taste of grace. Having received this grace, I became thankful and appreciative.

The idea of being a "nobody" does not sit well with the American culture. It is a label to be avoided at all costs. It is synonymous with being a loser, and no one wants to be a loser. To feel there is nothing we can do to improve our situation is frightening, especially if we look at it from the perspective that we have to do everything ourselves. Instead, if we believe that there is a power greater than us, a power that we can tap into that will guide our next steps, then the idea of doing nothing becomes more appealing. In this sense, doing nothing on the physical plane makes way for doing a great deal on the mental, emotional, and spiritual planes.

Doing nothing can be equated with waiting. In describing Apostle Paul's path, Charles Swindoll reminds us that, "Exceptional work is preceded by extended waiting."[28] We are a people who hate to wait. Road rage exists, not because we are kind and patient, but because we want what we want and we want it now. To do nothing is to practice patience and exercise trust. So, when the bases are loaded in relation to your life situation, instead of swinging for the fence on the first pitch in an effort to hit a grand slam, why not feel the intensity of the energy around you, and as you hold the bat up above your shoulder, just watch the ball come to you? See it travel from the pitcher's glove, and then hide from you as the windup proceeds. As it leaves the pitcher's hand, maybe you can begin to see its threads. It may spin, dip, or move away from or toward you. Listen for the "pop" as the ball hits the catcher's mitt, then take a deep breath and savor the moment.

There are choices in life. We have the freedom to make up our own minds on how we view our world. We can choose the hard way, which for most of us would seem to be the physicist's study of the subject of nothing. The easy way, however, can be practiced by virtually anyone. But in reality, is the easy way really so easy? Our natural inclination toward impatience and restlessness would have us believe that it's not. But with practice, stilling oneself will become increasingly less challenging, until finally, it's as effortless as breathing in and out. You owe it to yourself to begin taking steps toward grace. I challenge you to make time to intentionally sit and do nothing.

Notes: The Art of Doing Nothing

1. Martin, Philip. *The Zen Path through Depression.* (San Francisco, Harper Collins, 2000), p. 1.
2. Everything you ever wanted to know about how we spend our time, excluding anything to do with sex, can be found at the American Time Use Survey Summary at: http://www.bls.gov/TUS.
3. Ibid.
4. Ibid.
5. Ibid.
6. Ibid.
7. 2 Thessalonians 3:6 is quoted from the New International Version Bible found at BibleGateway.com
8. Iyengar, B.K.S. *Light on Yoga.* (New York, Schocken Books, 1979), pp. 422-424.
9. Beales, Gerald, *The Biography of Thomas Alva Edison.* http://www.thomasedison.com/biog.htm.
10. Shukla, Madhukar. *The Creative Muse: Stories of Creativity and Innovation.* http://www.geocities.com/madhukar_shukla/crebook/23.html.
11. Cruz, Richard. *Sleep Paralysis: REM and the "I Function."* This paper was written by a student for a course at Bryn Mawr College and is not to be considered as an authoritative work on the subject. http://serendip.brynmawr.edu/bb/neuro/neuro00/web2/Cruz.html.
12. More information on the stages of sleep can be found at: Infoaging.org: http://www.infoaging.org/l-sleep-01-stages.html.
13. See Psychology World. *Stages of Sleep* at: http://web.umr.edu/~psyworld/sleep_stages.htm.
14. For a mathematical description of a vacuum see: Mathematical Supplement H, *Physics of the Vacuum,* http://www.colorado.edu/philosophy/vstenger/Nothing/H_PhysVac.pdf.
15. Bayles, Jerry, E. *The Vector Magnetic Potential and A Schrodinger Wave Equation Solution for Electrogravational Mechanics.* This complex article filled with physics and calculus can be found at: http://www.electrogravity.com/AVECWAVE/AVecWave.pdf.
16. A full explanation of eigenvalues and their applications can be found at: http://mathworld.wolfram.com/Eigenvalue.html.
17. See *Matrix Diagonalization* – From MathWorld at: http://mathworld.wolfram.com/MatrixDiagonalization.html.
18. Barrow, John, D. *The Book of Nothing: Vacuums, Voids, and the Latest Ideas about the Origins of the Universe.* (New York, Pantheon Books, 2000), pp. 12-48.
19. Ibid.
20. Ibid.

21. Yancey, Philip. *What's So Amazing About Grace?* (Grand Rapids, Michigan, Zondervan Publishing, 1997), p. 30.

22. Merriam-Webster Online Dictionary at: http://www.m-w.com/dictionary/grace.

23. For more information on American's beliefs in God, heaven, angels, UFOs, astrology, reincarnation, and witches, see: *FOX News Poll* at: http://www.foxnews.com/story0,2933,99945,00.html.

24. See Religious Tolerance.org. Comparing U.S. Religious Beliefs with other "Christian Countries."

25. Swindoll, Charles, R. *Paul: A Man of Grace and Grit.* (Nashville, Tennessee, The W Publishing Group, 2002), pp. 1-16.

26. Ibid, p. 22.

27. Ibid, p. 52.

28. Ibid, p. 79.

CHAPTER 9

Joy 4 You

The "vanity" license plate reads, "Joy 4 You." Just a few years ago, it was a true vanity plate, as it had her name on it followed by the number 1. What happened in this person's life to bring about this change of focus Where she once was the center of her own world, she now has expanded her consciousness to become a harbinger of joy.

What exactly is joy? It is another one of those words that we all know superficially, but never take the time to examine where it truly fits into how we view our world and the relationships that we value. Many of the books we read today try to explain what joy is by example. This is an effective way to convey the experience of joy, as we have all had our moments in the sun, but here we are looking for a way to go deeper into the concept so that we can come away with a working knowledge of joy.

One way to rekindle the feeling of joy in your life is to find an old photo album and search for a picture that your parents took when you were having a great time just being yourself. It may have been a picture of you at the park on a summer day. You were standing there posing for the picture in your shorts, t-shirt, and sneakers, and the look on your face and the gleam in your eyes lets everyone know that you couldn't have been more content. This is just the way kids are: happy to be where they are, doing what they are doing, with no conditions attached.

One of the benefits of living a life with more joy is that it will bring higher energy to your days. Mira Kirshenbaum tells us, in *The Emotional Energy Factor: The Secrets High-Energy People Use to Beat Emotional Fatigue*, that even Gandhi urged his followers to enjoy life. His belief, which stemmed from the writings found in the *Isavasya Upanishad*, was that the universe is basically good, and since we are part of this universe, we also share this basic goodness.[1] *The Upanishads* are teachings of Hindu philosophy. In these ancient Vedic doctrines, it is stated that, "there is a core of certainty which is essentially incommunicable except by a way of life. It is by a strictly personal effort that one can reach the truth."[2] And so it is with the understanding of joy. Until we begin to live a life of joy, we will not be in a position to reap the benefits of such living, and we will do so only after expending some effort.

When a person meditates, especially when one practices mantras (spiritual hymns), a connection is made with the universe. To sit and repeat the most popular mantra, "Om," one is affirming "the identity of the individual consciousness with the Absolute or Divine reality."[4] Understanding this concept allows us to accept the pain with the pleasure, the heartbreak with the victory, and the joy and the sorrow in our experiences. Our task here is to ferret out the conditions, or threads, that are needed to isolate the compartment of joy that we call our own. Examine it; take it out and play with it, and hopefully, in the process, allow it to occupy a larger space in our day.

Amelia Earhart Putman, the courageous pilot and the first female to fly across the Atlantic, wrote a poem entitled *Courage*. In it she expresses the mixed and opposing emotions that are experienced by all those who dare to be courageous. It goes like this:

Courage

Courage is the price which life exacts for granting peace.
The soul that knows it not, knows no release
From little things:
Knows not the livid loneliness of fear,
Nor mountain heights where bitter joy can hear
The sound of wings.

How can Life grant us boon of living, compensate
For dull grey ugliness and pregnant hate
Unless we dare
The soul's dominion? Each time we make a choice, we pay
With courage to behold the resistless day,
And count it fair.[5]

Life is innately complex, when even the discussion of the topic of joy is mixed with phrases like "dull, gray ugliness" and "pregnant hate." With all of this deep pondering and all of the woes and cares in the world, it is almost unnatural to consider the idea of joy.

Take a moment to review some of the disastrous events that have occurred around the world in the first decade of the 21st century alone. To make it easy for yourself, pick up the December 19, 2005 special issue of *Time Magazine,* review the section on *The Best Photos of the Year*, and remember what a wicked year it was for hundreds of thousands of people. As Richard Lacayo, the author of the accompanying article in Time Magazine, quotes Susan Sontag, she described what images and photos do for us in the following way: "Narrative can make us understand, photographs do something else: they haunt us."[6]

Many of the images display the destruction and suffering caused by hurricane Katrina, as it hit the Gulf Coast on August 29, 2005. The photos clearly show the devastation and fear that this natural disaster created. The dead bodies floating face down in the water bring about the surreal tone surrounding the disaster. These images show scenes that we usually pay money to see in the movie theater—not what we expect to see in our own neighborhoods.

Next, there was the October 8, 2005 earthquake that left 88,000 dead in Pakistan. The body of the young student, lying dead in the rubble that was his school, could have just as easily been you or me. In another photo showing eight men praying as they look upon the remains of their mosque, I see great faith that their God will provide for them even in the wake of such destruction. Then there was the tsunami that claimed the lives of over 230,000 people in twelve countries, not to mention the number of individuals that it left homeless. Like you and I, they were living their lives the best they knew how, yet their hopes, dreams, relationships, and existences were cut short by a natural disaster.

Even more recently, all of the world was shocked as we viewed in real-time the devastation caused by the magnitude 9 earthquake and resultant tsunami that hit Japan. This disaster left over 350,000 people homeless and over 10,000 dead. The earthquake was so strong that it mangled railroad tracks, moved houses off their foundations, shifted the earth on its axis, and actually moved the main island of Japan by as much as 13 feet. To review these incredible pictures and read the associated stories, enter the following into your web browser: *Japan Tsunami: 20 Unforgettable Pictures - National Geographic.*

Where is the joy in all of these pictures? There is none. As the Bible tells us, there is a season for everything. For those whose lives were taken by these devastating events, they no longer have a voice to share with us, but the words, ideas, and feelings that we can experience from all of this seemingly senseless loss are significant. Through such extreme loss, we can begin to change the way we think about our lives and make minor, and sometimes major, changes in our priorities.

We all know that life is short, but we do not live like we believe this. The first major shift toward living like our days are limited occurred after 9/11. We, as a society, began to rearrange our priorities. Even in the medical profession, many of the newly trained physicians coming out of their residencies and fellowships are no longer totally willing to give up their lives to the profession, as was expected in the past. The day of the doctor as the hero is over, and to that I say, "Hallelujah."

New docs want to spend time with their young families. They want to spend quality time with their spouses. Many no longer want to follow the path of long on-calls eight or nine times a month, and work schedules that keep them on call from 8 a.m. Friday morning until 7 or 8 p.m. Monday. They now understand that such workloads take their toll on everyone around them, from the patients they see, the staff they work with, to the wife and children at home. They are not blind, and are very aware of the physician divorce and suicide rates. It appears that Americans are waking up, and because of this, I see more joy in everyone's future.

When something is off in our lives, we get messages to that effect. When we choose not to listen to the messages, they get louder and more obvious. These natural disasters can be viewed as messages to all of us, and I think we are beginning to listen.

One way to generate more joy in our lives is to abandon envy and jealousy. We all possess the freedom of choice when it comes to where we focus our thoughts. If we choose to dwell on the idea of what others have and what we are lacking, whether intentionally or out of ignorance, then we will suffer and live in a joyless state. If, on the other hand, we choose to be happy concerning what others have, then such an attitude brings more joy our way. The beauty of this is that, when we become aware and decide to change our attitude it, is possible to do so. It will take a great deal of work to retrain the way we think, and there will be setbacks, but over time things will look brighter.

Many times we may think about the wealth that others possess, but rarely do we ever think about the wealth they have to maintain to keep their worlds spinning in the same orbits day in and day out. A big home is an awesome thing to look at from the street, but we don't stop to think about the cost of yearly taxes, or lawn maintenance, or the cost of painting every few years. Next time you go by a big house and wonder what it is like to live there, take a moment to thank that person for their tax dollars, and consider how that money contributes to the services that you receive. Sometimes a simple creative twist in the way we see things is enough to quell our envy and turn our attitude toward rejoicing.

As Thubten Chodron tells us in *Working with Anger*, "rejoicing is an attitude that appreciates and enjoys others' happiness, talents, wealth, knowledge, skills, and virtue."[6]

The great thing about joy is that it is free. We do not have to pay a dime for it and it is available to us twenty-four hours a day. The hard part is that, in order to know joy, we have to drop all of the ego stuff that we carry around that keeps us feeling cheated or hurt. This is the freedom that comes with the understanding that the decision is ours to make, and no other individual or group of individuals has the power to keep us from joy unless we let them. If you currently find yourself in a position where you believe that your joy is dependent on others, then there is a great deal of work to be done. Because we are so comfortable in our thought patterns, even though they may be harmful to us and our loved ones, we resist changing our thinking. Not only do we make excuses as to why we are the way we are, but we adamantly hold on to images of past hurts and believe that we are doomed to repeat the mistakes.

How do we change such long-held beliefs? One of the most effective ways is to begin to appreciate all that we have right now. Instead of telling ourselves that we will be happy when our house is paid for or when we retire, it is liberating to be thankful for our current circumstances, no matter how difficult they may appear. Even in our troubles, we should be thankful. We can show gratitude for the fact that we were given such a difficult challenge in the first place in that facing such adversity, even though the outcome may be unknown, we will come away with greater knowledge and understanding about our lives and the world. We are being trusted to get though all of our difficulties, and we will get though them. It is just so much easier and more pleasant when we have the capacity to trust right from the get-go. Even if we are untrusting at the present time, we can learn to develop trust—trust in God or the universe, trust in ourselves, and trust in others.

Joy and excitement go hand-in-hand. To the uninformed, the energy of excitement is easily confused with fear. The sweaty palms, the racing heart, and the increased alertness all keep us on our toes, but when we tell ourselves that we are going to label these feelings as excitement and not cower in fear over what we are feeling, we find that the energy of excitement helps us to perform better than we expected.

When is the last time you got excited over your perceived problems? The idea of thinking this way would almost seem counterintuitive, but when we are excited, we see things in a totally different way than when we are in a state of fear. Fear, with its power to paralyze, will keep us from action, whereas excitement charges us with anticipation of what will come our way next, allowing us to see more options and potential in our situations.

An effective way to start to develop the view that our problems and roadblocks can actually be a source of excitement is to understand and live what the Buddha called the Five Remembrances. As explained by Thich Nhat Hanh, they include the following:

> 1. I am of the nature to grow old. There is no way to escape growing old.
> 2. I am of the nature to have ill health. There is no way to escape ill health.
> 3. I am of the nature to die. There is no way to escape death.
> 4. All that is dear to me and everyone I love are of the nature to change. There is no way to escape being separated from them.
> 5. My actions are my only true belongings. I cannot escape the consequences of my actions. My actions are the ground upon which I stand.[7]

Acting with these thoughts in mind will help us to appreciate whatever comes our way, as we will understand that even what we perceive as the worst experience of our lives is a temporary condition. We prolong our suffering when we allow the uncontrolled mind to wander off into the future while we are going through a difficult period. It is as if the mind has no idea of the present, and because of fear, it closes in on itself and sees an eternity of darkness, pain, lack, and joylessness. Like a little child who thinks everything is about him or her, an untrained mind will bring us deeper into a state of distress and misery.

On the other hand, when we recite the Five Remembrances, we remind ourselves that there is balance in life. We are alive right now, we are with our loved ones, and we do get sick, but for most of us sickness is temporary, then we feel better. We may be getting older, but we have the choice to do so gracefully. We give ourselves the option to rejoice at our current lot in life, even though, at times, our egos try to convince us that the life we have is inadequate.

Remembering our impermanence and the non-lasting nature of everything acts as a soothing salve that eases the pain associated with loss and change.

The next time you feel bothered by an interruption—be it by your child, spouse, co-worker, or a stranger on the street—instead of looking at it as an intrusion on your time, think of it as a honor that this other individual had the desire to come to you and seek your attention. This idea alone is enough to generate joy in your life multiple times a day, as the phone is always ringing and others have needs with which we may assist.

The question comes up as to how one experiences joy when dealing with the issue of chronic pain. According to the *Concise Encyclopedia of Pain Psychology,* chronic pain lasts six months or longer affects more than 20 percent of the population, and is typically distinguished from acute pain based on temporal characteristics. In contrast to acute pain, it is difficult to determine the inciting stimulus in chronic pain, since it no longer serves an adaptive role as a warning signal. As well, psychological factors play a greater role where chronic pain is concerned.[8] Once chronic pain sets in, pain receptors and nervous tissues become hyper-activated, and an individual will experience amplification of their pain. An article written by Min Zhuo, Ph.D., published in the journal *Neuron,* demonstrated that this supercharged pain phenomenon is due to the presence of two proteins in the brain: adenylyl cyclase 1 and 8. These proteins are found primarily in the anterior cingulated cortex - that portion of the brain that is important for feeling pain.[9]

Until scientists are able to develop drugs that will inhibit the function of the above mentioned proteins, those suffering from chronic pain are left to use standard medications such as acetaminophen, and NSAID's like Motrin, Aleve, and Celebrex, with their potential gastrointestinal side effects and possible cardiac side effects. Celebrex, like Vioxx, is a COX-2 inhibitor. It will be a long time before anyone forgets the heart problems caused by Vioxx. Many families, lawyers, and pharmaceutical companies will be dealing with issues surrounding this drug for years to come. When the above class of drugs are no longer effective in controlling pain, doctors move to the narcotic analgesics such as hydrocodone (Lortab, Vicodin, Tylenol #3 and #4), morphine, hydromorphone (Dilaudid), and most recently, fentanyl (Duragesic). When these high-powered drugs do not control pain, or when their side effects negatively affect quality of life, then folks are left with alternative forms of therapy, that is, if physicians, friends, or self- study brings this to their attention. This is where mind-body medicine has its greatest potential usefulness, but part of the problem is getting individuals to actually sit down and make the effort to give mindfulness a try.

In almost all things in life, it is our attitude that shapes our perceptions, and fortunately attitudes are open to change. Individuals who suffer from chronic pain generally tend to catastrophize, or imagine things are worse than they really are. This is not to minimize their pain, but it is a well known risk factor for developing chronic pain. Whether this kind of thinking is innate or a learned trait is a matter of question. The meat of the matter is that we all have choices. We can consciously choose to no longer be afraid of pain or afraid of whatever it is that is holding us back. To rethink and reorganize our thoughts will take effort, but it is better to expend the energy that will bring on some relief in the future than it is to live in a state of continual dread.

All during the course of our lives, we dread one thing after another. As children, we dread going to school. We especially dreaded the days when we had quizzes or tests. We then dread mowing the lawn or doing the dishes. Then once we start a job, after the initial excitement of being hired and receiving the first few paychecks, we dread going to work. It appears that our expectations lead us down the road of discontent. If, instead of feeling upset when things do not pan out the way we had wished for, we choose to be thankful for whatever unfolds and give up our need to feel that everything has to be the way we want it, we remove ourselves from the place of suffering.

To live in a state of joy, it is almost necessary to drop all ideas of who we think we are; release all images of why we believe we are the way we are, and take on the attitude that we are created new in each moment. In that creative process there is joy and wonder. Even if we create conditions that we later feel are no longer right for us, we can still assume the attitude that we can recreate what we think we want now. Life is indeed a paradox and is made up of opposites. In readings on the Tao (Chinese for "the way of life"), the concept of *yin-yang* developed around the third century BC. In the same manner, it is easy to understand that we cannot experience joy without sadness, and to think that we could be continually joyous is to be out of touch with reality.

Those beliefs and attitudes that keep us wasting our energies foolishly are obstacles to joy. We have the potential to keep our thoughts in one place at a time. This is so, even though we think we are being efficient in our abilities to multitask. Even with such skilled behavior, the brain is only capable of acting on one thought at a time. Some of the thoughts may be unclear or divided, but we can only focus on one at a time. In order to make way for joy, we need to ask ourselves what needs to be dropped so that joy and its attendant feelings and emotions can enter into our consciousness. How do we become more aware of the thoughts that bring us joy?

We can't smile and frown simultaneously. In order to smile we need to drop the frown, drop the thought patterns that brought on the frown, replace them with thoughts of joy and satisfaction, and then a smile will result. Anger is one of the most common emotions that blocks our joy. Anger is ubiquitous; it is easy to arouse in the unwatched or unexamined mind. It layers itself with each hurt, slight, or biting word. What damage it does to those who hold on to it and make it their constant companion. What pain it causes in those who rely on it to get them by. Unresolved anger leads to death - death in the emotional body, mental body, spiritual body, and at times, the physical body.

The difficulty with anger is that when it is allowed to build and go on unchecked, it comes to a level where it becomes so overwhelming that to penetrate it is very difficult. Anger can become a protective shell that allows no good thing to come in or go out. Turbulence, negative feelings, and worse case scenarios mumble and jumble to occupy consciousness. No wonder there is no room for joy. The recognition and acknowledgement of anger is a step by step process. Just as when a flower petal opens, it does so in progressive stages. It doesn't just burst open. It requires a slow, persistent approach to come to grips with anger. It's hot. It burns. It is painful and is not much fun to deal with. With enough rain and sunlight, the flower will blossom, and so will joy come to fruition if we dig up the hard frozen ground where the source and hidden reactions of anger are hidden.

To say that I am angry is to take the first step in the process of resolution of our anger. For now, it is not necessary to be concerned with the "why" of the anger. Getting over the denial of this emotion takes a change in the way we see ourselves. We have to be comfortable with the fact that anger is a legitimate feeling and that when we experience strong feelings of anger, we are not bad or unlovable. We get into trouble when we try to bury the anger in that over time, we lose sight of the inciting event and eventually we just go around feeling angry all of the time.

Notice how easy it is for thoughts to jump toward the hurts of the past. We hold images of others who have hurt us and end up blaming them for our current troubles. Look closely at this and see if you can take this particular person out of the picture. It will take effort to let their image and energy slide into the background, but as your efforts become more effective, as you ease your mental clasp of this "evil-doer," notice what is left behind to deal with. What is left behind is you.

When did you allow your thoughts and feelings to project away from yourself and give your power to others? Who comes to mind when you ask yourself this question? Once this person or situation is identified, rise up your courage and tell yourself not to be afraid, and take that person into yourself and engulf them with all of the love you can muster today. Don't worry if you cannot release these images in one attempt. You have started the process; it will keep moving along toward resolution as long as you keep coming back to it. Do not look for an end to the process, but instead realize that the good, the bad, the ups and downs, and the neutral aspects are all part of the life process.

Allow the ropes that keep you bound in your current thought process to fall to the ground so that you and your loved one's can experience freedom. Claim your joy and embrace it. Do not allow anger to keep hanging on. See it, feel what you can of it, then drop it as much as possible, thus making room for perfect joy. Celebrate your rediscovery of joy.

Other obstacles to joy are envy and jealousy. When we feel insecure and unsure of our own capabilities, it is natural to look around and notice what others have that we lack. Keeping our thoughts on the idea of lack is the surest way to stay in a state of need. At these times, it is possible to give thanks for what we have. Most of us can see; we have good eyesight and clear vision. But do we really see our daily gifts? With our minds all wrapped up in what we don't have, we lose sight of what we do have now.

We can see the blue sky, but how many times do we simply look up to appreciate the expansiveness of our sky above? It is our sky to enjoy. No one owns it and it is part of what has been given to us to marvel at. We have ears; they too, like our eyes, are incredibly tuned instruments that allow the recognition of wonder. How many times have we heard a voice and thought, "Oh God, not them?" Instead of judging who a person is, why not listen to their voice and not react to what we think we hear in their attitude; find joy in the fact that another voice, for whatever reason, wants to speak with you. You are being recognized by another. This is a gift that we too often fail to acknowledge. Because we create our own dysfunction, we can also create joy and make room for greater degrees of it daily. Make the conscious decision to open the gateway for more joy to enter into your life today, and it will happen.

Notes: Joy 4 You

1. Kirshenbaum, Mira. *The Emotional Energy Factor: The Secrets High-Energy People Use to Beat Emotional Fatigue.* New York: Delacorte Press, 2003, pp. 62-63.

2. There are four Vedas, each consisting of four parts: the mantra sections (samhita or hymns), the ritualistic teachings (brahmana), the theological sections (aranyaka), and the philosophical sections (Upanishads). For more information on the Upanishads and Vedas see: *The Hindu Universe* at http://www.hindunet.org/upanishads/.

3. Ibid.

4. The poem *Courage* is quoted from *Fun Facts*, The Amelia Earhart Museum, http://www.ameliaearhartmuseum.org/funfact1.htm.

5. The photos described can be viewed in *Time*: Special Issue, December 19, 2005, pp. 77-133.

6. Chodron, Thubten. *Working with Anger.* Ithaca: Snow Lion Publications, 2001, p. 123-124.

7. Thich Nhat Hanh. *The Heart of the Buddha's Teaching: Transforming Suffering into Peace, Joy, and Liberation.* New York: Broadway Books, 1998, pp. 121-130.

8. Fillingim, Roger, B. *Concise Encyclopedia of Pain Psychology.* New York: Haworth Press, 2005, p. 21.

9. Wei F, Chang-Shen Q, Kim SJ, Muglia L, Maas JW Jr., Pineda W, Xu HM, Chen ZF, Storm DR, Muglia LJ, Zhuo M. "Genetic elimination of behavioral sensitization in mice lacking calmodulin-stimulated adenyl cyclases." *Neuron*, November 14, 2002, Vol. 36, pp. 713-726.

SUMMARY

Discover the Joy of Good Health

Having read *Discover the Joy of Good Health,* you have been introduced to the powerful yet simple concept of expressing a genuine smile and how difficulty in its expression can indicate the presence of unprocessed anger, fear or frustration. The exercise of examining an earlier picture of yourself and reconnecting with the child you were can go a long way toward self-healing. Recalling the wonder and joy that felt ever-present allows one to soften back into the present without displaying the rough edges that life's bumpy road ingrained into your psyche.

Also in chapter one, we discussed the development of a life timeline with insertion of associated feelings, emotions, and expectations at that particular time. This exercise allowed the reader to examine belief systems that were developed in early childhood, and that may have stunted the development of personal growth. Once examined in this safe way, beliefs that needed adjustment could be changed as desired.

The concept of "doing nothing" in a difficult situation was presented, as was the need to move out of survival mode with the idea of just getting by. We reviewed the idea that seeing clearly is more important to the attainment of happiness than the acquisition of material things.

In chapter two, the importance of focus was brought to the forefront. Just as a laser focuses light to do its work, as we focus our intention and thought on a desired goal, be it physical, mental, or spiritual, we find manifestation comes with less effort. The understanding of the concept of mirroring each other showed us how to move away from negative influences and move toward more positive energy in order to tap into our creative spirits. Also discussed was the appreciation of connectedness and engagement with others, which allows for an inner shifting of consciousness, thus making us feel a part of something bigger than ourselves.

Questions about what it means to be patient were reviewed, as was the acceptance of shifting perspective to change a negative attitude toward a past injury, and how that change in attitude becomes the actual stepping-stone to inner freedom. As in the first chapter, examples of the idea of doing nothing showed us the benefits of reviewing and playing with potential outcomes before important decisions are made.

Chapter two also showed us how we are not our fears. Our reactions and expectations are a result of chemical and physiological reactions occurring in our brain. One of the driving points in this chapter is our ability to exercise trust and know that what the mind can do, it can also undo to our benefit.

In chapter three, the importance of practicing praise and the appreciation of self and others was stressed. In the realization of our own special abilities, we need not covet the gifts of others, but appreciate our contributions and those of others to the betterment of all. The importance of recognizing our dark side was presented, in that failure to do so can lead to self-hate and self-sabotage. The exploration and identification of our sub-personalities and their value in how they work together to dictate our comfort levels in daily life. The idea of genuine praise was equated with caring and having a healthy sense of self-worth.

Chapter four, "Conditions We Live By," had to do with boundaries and how they are set during childhood. Once the realization occurs that much of our behavior is based on past conditioning, we can move ahead with greater mindfulness and act on real-time beliefs. The importance of allowing oneself to slow down in making difficult life changes was reviewed. In moving at a slower pace, we feel safe to open up space for new experiences and ways of feeling your fears; it is not easy, but it is doable with trust and gentleness.

The need to please others is a stumbling block that causes one to act on mixed messages, thus impeding progress and growth. In asking for what we want, being present, changing self-talk, expressing one's dreams, and setting goals, we realize the possibility of making our own thoughts and wishes priority, without guilt, while simultaneously respecting those of others. Chapter four also highlighted the importance of expecting the best, feeling genuinely, being grateful, giving to others, and the benefits of journaling.

In the next chapter, we learned about the study of compassion and how the first step to move in that direction is simple: we must make time for such study, making it a priority. It was shown that this work involves a search for internal and external motivating factors, the willingness to recognize suffering, and the coupling of this recognition with a desire to help relieve suffering. Knowing the right questions to ask from the outset is paramount to getting off to a good start. These questions were reviewed in depth. A ten-point, "How to Measure Compassion," questionnaire was presented that was intended to be used on a daily basis as a means of tracking progress. Methods for growth in generating compassion for the self and others were also presented in detail, as was the ubiquitous feeling of shame and how to extract oneself from its grip.

Chapter five also discusses the complex interplay of toxin-handlers: those who voluntarily shoulder the emotional burdens of co-workers. Contrasted with the insensitivity of hard-nosed managers and leaders who alienate their workforce by ignoring their frustrations, the empathy of the toxin-handler was shown to make for better morale in the workplace. However, as beneficial as the toxin-handler's role might be, the potential effects on their emotional and physical well-being could be devastating.

How we deal with change and the roles that patience and expectations play in accepting change was explored in chapter six. The results of failing to deal with change effectively were discussed, in that remaining insensitive to the early signs of change leads to one crisis after another. The knowledge involved in the practice of making conscious and unconscious choices that bring about change was discussed. The word pairs IS/IS NOT, AND/OR, SOME/ALL, BEFORE/AFTER, NOW/LATER, SAME/DIFFERENT were presented, and we discussed how their use helps to simplify the process of making choices and fostering the change that we desire.

Chapter seven focused on authority issues and how the need to control the masses over time has filtered down even to the present. This need for control affects each of us in different ways. Past councils, such as The Inquisition, put fear in the hearts of populations of nonconformists. Even today, people all over the world are controlled by governing parties where the good of the common man and woman are not top priorities. Bringing this concept closer to home, we see the negative effects of parents exerting excessive control over their children. This results in the unpreparedness and inability to make decisions as the child matures. They are instead set up to succumb to peer pressure or the wishes of others. It was further discussed that effective decision-making relies on one's ability to differentiate between what is real and what is imagined. We each have to decide on our degree of compliance when it comes to societal expectations, knowing that a certain degree is necessary and healthy.

Other main topics found in chapter seven dealt with the issues of trust versus mistrust, and learning to listen to our own inner voices. Questions posed on this topic were meant to help readers move toward developing the inner wisdom that will never fail them.

As we moved on to chapter eight, we examined the paradoxical idea of "doing nothing" in order to get what we need and want. Especially helpful during states of mental depression, a conscious focus on "nothingness" helps to quiet psychological and emotional noise, which so often goes unseen by the outside world. This state is equated to the winter of our lives, and when spring comes around again, there is new life. This chapter also revealed the day-to-day activities of the typical American, as it relates to the importance and rejuvenating effects of carving out time for daily reflection. It was explained how, by doing nothing for short periods of time, we learn to appreciate the connectedness and relationships we have with others. In the act of doing nothing, we reap the reward of moving from the unreal images of the imagination to the real.

We concluded with an in-depth discussion about grace and how, in our culture, we have to make a conscious effort to accept the idea and gift of grace. Since we believe that we have to do it all—all of the time—we will eventually stumble and blame ourselves for the failure, instead of looking to a higher power for help. The chapter ends with the insights gained in that, as we do nothing, what we are really doing is practicing patience and feeling the life force within and all around us.

The final chapter covered the topic of joy and how we can rekindle joy in our daily lives. Even in the face of trials, we can choose to concentrate on joy by making a conscious decision to do so. Yes—it can be that easy, and no—it has no relationship to living in denial. It is simply a matter of where we choose to place our attention. In a joyous state, we will naturally express more gratitude. Joy has to do with sharing, and if you think about it, what we all really want to do is to share our ideas and our lives with others. It is what makes us complete. It is the past rejections that we must get over in order to feel joy again.

In working with our emotions, feelings, and behaviors, we do have to realize that there is a season for everything under the sun. Learning to be patient, grateful, and compassionate will bring inner peace and allow us all to be more effective and comfortable with what we have to work with. Recall always: We have choices, and life will go much smoother when we begin to *Discover the Joy of Good Health*.

John Inzerillo, M.D.

John Inzerillo, M.D. is a board certified medical oncologist. He has practiced state-of-the-art oncology in eastern North Carolina for nineteen years. He appreciates his patient's willingness to enter into clinical trial research treatments when appropriate. Among his strengths is his background in dealing with patient's associated stress in relation to their respective diagnoses. Over the past three years, Dr. Inzerillo has has had the opportunity to share this knowledge with oncology health care workers including other oncology physicians, oncology nurses, office managers, and front office staff. This has been possible through a program offered by Eli Lilly Pharmaceuticals. Topics of discussion have included the following: Dealing with the Difficult Patient, Dealing with Loss and Grief, Difficult Discussions in Late-Stage Cancer Care, and Helping Patients Transition into Survivorship.

With an interest in stress management that goes back to his teenage years, he has followed the writings of such authors as Herbert Benson M.D., Thomas Moore (*Care of the Soul*), and Jon Kabat-Zinn (*Full Catastrophe Living, Wherever You Go there You Are*). His interests in the human stress response and how to deal with it led him into the study of Hatha Yoga. He has shared this knowledge with cancer survivors over the years through weekly yoga instruction. His personal yoga practice continues to this day.

With all of the distressful news with which we are bombarded on a daily basis, Dr. Inzerillo wanted to take pen to paper and give readers restorative and positive ideas upon which to dwell. These are ideas and thoughts that he tries to incorporate daily into his life.

Living in a quiet, North Carolina town on the Pamlico River, he enjoys his time with his wife of twenty years, and with his two sons, whom he considers his greatest gifts.

More great books from Humanics Publishing to stimulate your thinking. Available at your local bookstore or visit www.humanicspub.com.

Passion Beyond Pain
As our population ages there will be increasing numbers of individuals who will be confronted with chronic pain conditions, frailty, and the depression associated with these states of being. There is an urgent and ever increasing need to recognize these symptoms and build a medical community that will successfully and ably deal with these issues. Passion Beyond Pain is another brick in the wall that will assist all of us to care for each other to the best of our abilities as our compassion and understanding matures.
PAPERBACK   9780893344542 $18.95

The Mental Diet
Tony Leggett has helped thousands of people around the world, his profound teachings can help change your life in every area too. Tony wants to help you with your journey. He is passionate about his seven day program, and ready to help you break through the fear that is holding you back. As you will read in this book, he too, has suffered and has known fear. He too, thought that there was no way to change his life. But he found that faith and persistence are the antidote to fear.
PAPERBACK   9780893348892 $14.95

The Tao of Calm
The Tao of Calm is for those seekers of peace in the activities of daily life: Harried parents, pressured office workers, teachers, students, and others who feel that there is never enough time for the desired calm to balance their busy lives. These 81 meditations are modeled after the writing of the Chinese philosopher, Lao Tzu, whose timeless teachings in the book, Tao Te Ching, have survived through the years. In The Tao of Calm, Dr. Pamela Metz stays true to the spirit and structure of the Tao Te Ching while creating a guide for the readers to find a path of calmness in their lives. The author recognizes that many of us live lives of pressure, anxiety and stress, with little tie for centering and reflection. In this book, the poetic images of water, mountains, sky and earth evoke places of inner and outer calm.
PAPERBACK   0893343692 $17.95

Balance of Body Balance of Mind
Ancient Buddhist meditations and modern Western somatic therapy are united by their healing capabilities in this fascinating book. Both philosophies recognize that a structurally balanced human body is the key to a mentally and emotionally balanced human mind. The beautiful simplicity of the healing techniques and explanations detailed within will ensure that you attain the spiritual and physical balance needed to create an optimum environment for yourself.
PAPERBACK   0893341630 $16.95